'This book creates ready access to multi-family therapy (MFT) which is at once the most challenging and the most rewarding of psychological therapies. The book catapults readers to the "sweet spot" for helping members of family groups re-acquire social understanding in the contexts where it matters most – collaborating with other families, supporting and being supported in equal measure.'

Prof. P. Fonagy, *University College London*

'The authors draw on the wealth of their own pioneering work developing intensive forms of MFT for various problems, as well as an in-depth knowledge of the literature, making the book a veritable MFT compendium. The book is both a great cover-to-cover read, as well as a useful reference book to return to when seeking inspiration for creative MFT activities or some problem-solving clinical wisdom.'

Prof. I. Eisler, *Institute of Psychiatry London*

'This book by internationally acclaimed MFT expert Dr. Eia Asen and his colleagues is the most comprehensive guide to creating, implementing and evaluating multi-family therapy. It should be a core text for any graduate course in mental health disciplines, as MFT is the most efficient, cost-effective approach to working with troubled families and to building family-based communities of support.'

Prof. P. Fraenkel, *The City College of the City University of New York*

W0113782

Systemic Multi-Family Therapy

This book provides a pragmatic guide to multi-family therapy (MFT), as employed in a variety of different settings: health, social care and education.

Bringing six to eight families together to work on similar issues in MFT has become an increasingly successful intervention that encourages service user-participation and moves towards a more patient- and family-centred care. This text describes the concepts, therapeutic stances, interventions and techniques of MFT, bringing together all the major recent developments in the field. Specific topics covered include how to engage families in working together with up to eight families with similar issues and problems, how to set up and conduct multi-family groups and how to evaluate and develop interventions. The book covers working with and across diverse cultures, conditions and problems and includes a chapter on different MFT exercises, activities and games.

Systemic Multi-Family Therapy is written for a range of practitioners, including psychotherapists, psychologists, psychiatrists, group therapists and family therapists, and will also be relevant for most professionals working in social care and schools.

Eia Asen, MD, Consultant Psychiatrist, Anna Freud Centre London; Visiting Professor, University College London. Previously Consultant Child and Adolescent Psychiatrist and Clinical Director, Marlborough Family Service London (NHS).

Emma Morris, DClinPsy, Consultant Clinical Psychologist, Head of Psychological Therapy Innovation, Anna Freud Centre, London. Director of the Multi-Family Project. Previously Clinical Psychologist, Marlborough Family Service, London (NHS).

Noël Pommepuy, MD, Child and Adolescent Psychiatrist, Head of Child and Adolescent Department, Ville-Evrard Hospital, Neuilly-sur-Marne (France). MFT trainer, Aprtf Paris.

Systemic Multi-Family Therapy

Concepts and Interventions

Eia Asen, Emma Morris and Noël Pommepuy

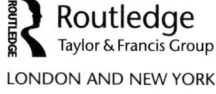
Routledge
Taylor & Francis Group

LONDON AND NEW YORK

Designed cover image: Patu Tifinger

First published 2025
by Routledge
4 Park Square, Milton Park, Abingdon, Oxon OX14 4RN

and by Routledge
605 Third Avenue, New York, NY 10158

Routledge is an imprint of the Taylor & Francis Group, an informa business

British Library Cataloguing-in-Publication Data
A catalogue record for this book is available from the British Library

ISBN: 9781032580760 (hbk)
ISBN: 9781032580746 (pbk)
ISBN: 9781003442424 (ebk)

DOI: 10.4324/9781003442424

Typeset in Times New Roman
by Apex CoVantage, LLC

Contents

Preface

In this book we describe the principles and aims of systemic MFT and its many techniques and applications in the different fields of mental health, social care and education. Systemic MFT is, above all, used in work with children, adolescents and their families. The book is essentially written for therapists, psychologists, social workers, teachers, psychiatrists and other disciplines that focus on improving the mental health of families and their members. We have chosen to refer to professionals undertaking MFT as 'MFT practitioners' or merely 'practitioners' rather than as 'therapists', 'clinicians', 'MFT coaches' or 'MFT workers'.

A brief overview of structure and content of the book may be helpful to readers. In Chapter 1 we review the diverse inspirations that have led to the development of systemic MFT and how different concepts are influencing its current practices. It is not usual in books of this nature to review the evidence base for a specific approach in the second chapter and to outline how to evaluate MFT projects. We have done so to emphasize the importance of critically examining the approach and encourage practitioners to think about doing so even before they embark on a new project, highlighting the importance of demonstrating that what one does actually works and that there is an ongoing commitment to learning from feedback.

In Chapter 3 we introduce some basic systemic techniques that can be adapted to multi-family work. One particular aspect of our MFT approach is the emphasis on promoting (more) effective mentalizing, and this is explained in some detail in Chapter 4. The subsequent chapter explains how to set up MFT projects and how to manage the initial work. A central part of our book is Chapter 6, in which we describe the many different exercises and games, which we term 'activities', that enrich MFT work. We do so by providing 'instructions' which we have framed in direct speech to make them more user friendly. These are only suggestions, and it is of course left to each MFT practitioner to find their own words for introducing a specific MFT activity. Throughout the book we mention and refer to many of the activities, and these are marked in italics and listed in three sub-sections in alphabetical order.

Chapter 7 looks at how practitioners can engage with culture and diversity, how to address and manage discriminatory behaviours 'head on' and to reflect their own cultural identity may contribute to group dynamics. The three subsequent sections of the book – Chapters 8, 9 and 10 – introduce specific MFT projects that can be applied in mental health, social services and education settings. In Chapter 11 we look at typical problematic issues one encounters during MFT work and provide some tips on how to manage these. The final chapter looks back on what MFT has achieved since its 'birth' almost eight decades ago and reflects on how it might develop over the next few decades.

This is not the first book written about the application of systemic ideas to MFT. Two previous publications (Asen et al., 2001; Asen & Scholz, 2010) have laid the foundation for this approach, and they contain some of the concepts and materials also referred to in this book. However, over the past 15 years, many new MFT projects have been initiated and much creativity has fuelled the work. We are grateful to many colleagues and friends who have inspired our work over the year, far too many to name them all. However, we will mention only a few here: Alan Cooklin, Michael Scholz, Ann Stevens, Derek Taylor, Ivan Eisler, Brenda McHugh, Neil Dawson, Katja Scholz, Maud Rix, Dietmar Selig, Petra Kiehl and Justine van Lawick. We have worked in close partnership with many talented teams in Europe, above all in England, Germany, Scandinavia, France, Poland, The Netherlands, Belgium, Switzerland and Italy. They have contributed many innovative ideas and practices and become much-valued members of our 'family' of MFT practitioners. Last not least, we want to thank the many many families who have tolerated our experimentation with the approach. We have learned more with and from them than we ever imagined. Without them this book would have never been written.

Chapter 1

Aims and basic principles

Therapeutic factors

MFT relies on the power of group work and the recognition that it is helpful for individuals experiencing emotional distress to discover that suffering is not an isolated experience, that other people do struggle with similar issues and that sharing these can lead to mutual support. Group-analytic psychotherapy utilized this dynamic when, in the 1940s in England, Sigmund Heinrich Foulkes and colleagues (Foulkes, 1948) convened 'closed' groups with up to eight patients who met weekly over many months with two therapists. These pioneers and subsequent group therapists identified various factors that influence positive change in group therapy, such as mutual support, imparting of information, interpersonal learning, imitative behaviour, constructive criticism and instillation of hope (Yalom & Leszcz, 1995).

These therapeutic factors are of course also relevant for MFT, but there is one major difference: it is not individuals who meet other individuals but whole families who meet other families and their members. Traditional group therapy is heavily dependent on verbal accounts of individual problems and relationship difficulties. By contrast, in MFT, family relationships and dynamics linked with the presenting problems can be 'seen' and addressed in a direct way. What is experienced and learned in the group setting can be taken home and practiced in the families' own 'real-life' contexts. Furthermore, MFT encourages the families' social networks of supporters to be indirectly, and sometimes directly, involved in the therapeutic process. Furthermore, unlike traditional group therapy, MFT supports families meeting outside the group context and creating a network of support away from the formal therapeutic work.

In the actual multi-family meetings, families become less defensive when they feel that they are 'all in the same boat together'. This leads to a greater degree of openness and to experimenting with being self-reflective in front of others. This is further enhanced when families and their individual members see themselves 'reflected' or mirrored in others, generating novel perspectives on seemingly 'familiar' dilemmas. With meeting new people, families and their individual members develop a form of positive 'curiosity' (Cecchin, 1987) about the minds of other group members. When families begin to voice their perceptions of others,

DOI: 10.4324/9781003442424-1

including critical ones, it is not at all uncommon that their comments or commentaries are better heard and understood than when very similar observations are made by professionals (Asen, 2002).

The aims and principles of MFT (see Box 1) are a mixture of action-oriented and reflective work, with families being actively encouraged to become consultants to other families, supporting each other while also reflecting on their own issues. MFT relies on the mechanisms of social and experiential learning and the related increase in self-esteem.

Box 1   Aims and objectives of MFT

Creating a sense of solidarity and reducing social isolation and stigmatization

Stimulating fresh perspectives and providing contexts where families can learn from each other

Strengthening reflectiveness in relation to one's own actions and situation via observing others

Encouraging mutual support and feedback and experimenting with cross-family exercises

Discovering and building on competencies, intensifying interactions and experiences and practicing new communications and behaviours in a safe space

Raising expectations and hopes for recovery

Contributing to solutions to other people's difficulties by sharing observations, suggestions and understandings

---

It is possible to practice MFT in a variety of contexts and locations, from sessional work lasting 2 hours once or twice a month, carried out in clinics, schools and various community settings, to much more intensive work in bespoke institutions such as day units for families (Asen et al., 1982). Here between six and eight families meet for 6 hours or longer on a daily or less frequent basis over months (see Chapter 9). There is no gold standard for the duration or frequency of sessions, as these are often determined by the specific needs of the group and institutional circumstances, such as humanpower or financial issues. The work can be carried out in closed as well as in open groups. In a closed group all families start and finish together. In open groups, families join and leave at different phases of the life of the group. In such a scenario the more experienced families can mentor new arrivals and provide hope and expertise from their positions of 'experts by experience'. As families take a more active role in the work, they become increasingly involved in the process of their own change, and this permits MFT practitioners to shift from a 'hands-on' to a 'hands-off' stance, moving increasingly to the periphery of what happens and eventually taking a 'back seat' (Asen, 2007).

Preparing families and their networks for MFT

Most people, professionals and families alike, will not know what MFT is, and anyone asked to participate in such work is likely to have understandable fears that they might be asked to 'air their dirty laundry in public' and that they might be criticized or misunderstood. Addressing these fears requires non-judgmental acceptance and sensitivity. In a preliminary single-family meeting with each family, the approach and its evidence base, advantages and disadvantages need to be explained patiently. Families can also meet 'graduate families' who have previously taken part in MFT and hear their accounts of the work. Prospective families are encouraged to bring their own supporters, extended family members, friends, even professionals, to such a first meeting. It is helpful to have a leaflet or a link to a website providing information about the group work that families can return to and consult. Such leaflets tend to be more effective if they are co-constructed or co-produced with families, parents *and* children, who have attended MFT groups previously, as they speak to the concerns they had prior to attending and therefore provide relevant information based on their experience of MFT. Families are more likely to engage in the group work if they are given a concrete account of what to expect, like a detailed overview of the structure of an MFT project or even a session-by-session description. Time then needs to be allowed for the information to be digested, and a second meeting can be scheduled some weeks later, with an informed and mutually agreed-upon decision then being made about participating in MFT or not. When a large professional network is already attached to a family, as tends to happen in most child protection cases, it is important to hold a formal professional network meeting at which the parents, their supporters and all currently involved professionals are also present. Here it can be negotiated what other interventions will continue, or not, while the family attends multi-family sessions. MFT is usually *not* a stand-alone approach but used in combination with other therapies and interventions.

Various MFT projects provide a 'taster' session for families (see Chapter 5) so they can meet other families and experience for themselves first-hand what the approach is like before making a commitment. Once a family has decided to commit themselves to participating in an MFT project, they meet all the other families for the first joint session. This is best kept as welcoming and informal as possible, with light refreshments being offered as the families arrive and engaging them in non-problem-oriented conversations. Family members are encouraged to introduce themselves without lengthy explanations or speeches, and this includes the practitioners! Once the formal part of the group starts, it is the practitioners' task to create a context that allows for participants to be able to begin to talk and to be heard. Initially this is best done in a large circle, with each family and its members in turn talking directly to the practitioners. This way of connecting with each family during the first session could be termed 'single family work in the presence of other families'. During this phase the practitioners are very central, and family members tend to address them rather than the members of other families whom, after all, they have never met before. Each family is spoken to in turn, and the practitioners try during these initial interactions to point out similarities, rather than differences, between the attending families.

The paradigm shift: From 'helped' to 'helper'

The majority of systemic MFT projects focus on work with children, young persons and their families, and these mostly take place in psychological and psychiatric services for children and adolescents, in social care and in schools. Professionals working in these services and institutions tend to adhere to the somewhat traditional concept of being a 'helper', and as the work often involves the temporary delegation of parental responsibility for the child/young person to staff and social workers, nurses, psychiatrists, psychologists, teachers and other professionals, there is a risk of them becoming temporary surrogate parents. This is the case especially when a child or young person is admitted to an inpatient unit, day hospital or residential social care setting, with the temptation for staff to become 'better parents' than the actual parents. This often-unconscious process may be accompanied by the parents' wish – reinforced by a currently pervasive consumer attitude – to get professional staff to 'fix' their child, or at least to act as some form of 'super-nanny'. It is especially at the beginning of MFT work and also in crisis situations that parents very quickly appeal for 'help' to the practitioners whom they want to see as experts. As systemic MFT emphasizes the agency of individuals and families and their own 'expertise', it places the responsibility on *them* for managing difficult situation and making changes rather than on the practitioners. However, refusing to be cast in the expert role is often not easy for practitioners, and comments such as 'I am an expert on MFT, but not on your children, you know them much better than I do' can begin to dispel this attitude. It is best followed up when the practitioners invite members of other families to provide their very own thoughts and ideas and to get them to have direct conversations with those parents. Sometimes it is best for there not to be any chairs available for the practitioners, so that they don't get stuck in a seat or 'fixed' place. Standing up to move and then walking between families or circling them, squatting or kneeling briefly in front of a family, and getting away after no more than 30 to 60 seconds can help to connect with a family or an individual whilst at the same time giving the message that not the practitioners but the actual families and their individual members are meant to help each other. This physical and mental mobility is a 'must' for MFT practitioners; they enact and alternate between being close and distant; they activate, warm up, focus, hand over responsibility to group members and then withdraw and on occasion even leave the room, thereby giving families the message that they can do 'their own thing'. Multi-family work requires multi-positional and 'roving' practitioners who are able to work 'on the move', shifting from 'doing' to merely 'observing' and then 'commenting' or questioning, and all this within very short time spans: practitioners' mindsets have to be flexible and adaptive.

Roles and functions of MFT practitioners

MFT practitioners have several different roles: they act as context makers and catalysts, making reactions and interactions possible that might otherwise not take place. For this to happen, as already observed, they cannot merely take a sitting-down position but have to be continuously 'on the move', building bridges between families. As soon as families or their individual members have established contact with one another, the practitioners can move away, signalling that families themselves need to 'get on with it' and 'with each other'. Once this process is set in motion, the practitioners can become increasingly less available and have less direct eye contact with individual group members. Instead, they continuously scan the room, with their eyes moving backwards and forwards all the time, signalling presence but at the same time de-emphasizing their own importance. The practitioners' increasing distancing tends to have the effect of activating group members to show more agency themselves. The continuous scanning and 'wandering' of the eyes can also be supported physically by the practitioners being on the move, as further described in Chapter 3.

MFT work cannot be carried out by just one practitioner; it requires a minimum of two professionals who have quite separate though complementary roles: one is in an 'active' and the other in an 'observing' role and position. These positions can be swapped so that each practitioner is for some part of the MFT session the *active* and for another part the *observing practitioner*. The observing practitioner follows the developing group process very closely and monitors all group members and their interactions with the active practitioner, in line with the truism that four eyes see more than two. The observing practitioner will only speak to the active one and not to group members directly, but loud enough for them to hear any conversations between the two practitioners. They do not sit next to each other but sit or stand far apart and across from each other, so that they can see one another and, if necessary, communicate via eye contact. The practitioners act transparently as equal partners who treat each other with respect, and this is evident to all the families. In other words, the practitioners try to collaborate and talk to each other in ways that well-functioning adults and parents might do. It is therefore quite possible that they will not always agree on how to deal with a specific issue, but they do so transparently and discuss their differences in front of the group. These discussions are not of a 'strategic' nature but always genuine and authentic. Roles and functions of MFT practitioners are summarized in Box 2.

Box 2   Roles and functions of MFT practitioners

- to prepare sessions
- to create a safe environment and containment for all families and their individual members

- to manage conflicts and discomfort of group members
- to connect families with families
- to facilitate MFT activities
- to facilitate reflections
- to generate transfer tasks
- to compile and keep records of sessions
- to assess and manage risk
- to be responsible for time keeping
- to be part of inter-session communications
- to keep in touch with professional networks
- to arrange supervision and/or intervision
- to evaluate outcomes of the work and invite feedback from families

Transfer of responsibility

In multi-family work with young children and their parents it is important that the latter be responsible throughout the session for their offspring. This is complicated when, for example, a once-weekly 2-hourly MFT session has to be integrated into an overall day-patient or in-patient/residential unit. Here the parents can only be responsible for their children during MFT, as for the rest of the time, professional staff care for the child 24 hours a day. In such scenarios the children or young people tend to have a 'home advantage', as the residential setting is temporarily their 'home'. By contrast, their parents may feel quite insecure and estranged, especially during the first MFT sessions. Some children therefore do not primarily relate to their parents at the beginning of an MFT group but rather to their 'surrogate carers', that is, the institution's professional staff. Parents can feel offended by this, which makes them feel even more insecure, but professional staff don't feel comfortable with this situation either. If such scenarios and transitions are not managed sensitively, professional staff will not know how they should behave if a child or young person relates primarily to them rather than to their own parents. To address these difficult situations, a ritual of handing over responsibility can take place, with the help of coloured glass balls or differently coloured friendship armbands: the child chooses one of these and hands them over to the parent for the duration of the MFT session. At the end, all balls and armbands are put back into a bag, which is then handed to a member of staff.

MFT as a context for doing other forms of systemic work

It is important to point out that MFT is not only a specific therapeutic tool or method but also a setting which permits the delivery of other systemic modalities, such as single-family work, couple work and work with just one individual, be that a parent or child. Convening therapeutic 'ad hoc' meetings with an individual for perhaps no longer than 10 minutes can be more meaningful and effective than a scheduled 50-minute formal psychotherapy session a few days later when heat and intensity of the perceived crisis has dissipated.

MFT is a challenge not only for families but also for clinicians. As the work is usually rather structured, with tight timetables and frequent transitions from one context to another, family members (and practitioners!) need to change or adapt their roles and functions continuously, often within the space of a few minutes! At one point they are members of a large group, a bit later they are 'merely' parents in charge of their children, then members of a parents or children only group, and shortly after one family amongst six or seven other families. These continuous context shifts generate a hothouse effect, increasing the pace of change, with staff and families being always 'on the move' and having to adopt multiple positions and changing perspectives. Positive group pressure further optimizes the effects of therapeutic interventions.

Confidentiality and consent issues

Confidentiality is an important issue in all forms of group therapy. Traditionally members are asked not to disclose anything that happens in sessions to the outside world. Yet this is quite an unrealistic request, particularly in MFT, as some of what happens in sessions is meant to be exported to the home context and also shared with their support network. Hence, a more realistic way to achieve confidentiality is to encourage members to discuss meaningful aspects of what happens in the sessions outside but without identifying details. Practitioners can at the very outset give practical examples of how one can do this and yet preserve the anonymity of other families and their members. Confidentiality cannot be guaranteed in MFT, but the point needs to be made that it is a shared responsibility and based on mutual trust and respect. Any rules and regulations for effective MFT work are best devised by the attending families themselves during the first or second session. However, some institutions insist on participating families signing a written contract. This can cover several issues and be sub-divided into what the family undertakes to agree on and what the MFT practitioners and their institution will insist on. The section of the contract for the family can cover the following issues:

- to be on time for all scheduled sessions;
- to notify the practitioners if not able to attend;
- to be respectful, non-violent and non-discriminatory to everyone attending MFT;
- not to attend MFT when under the influence of alcohol or drugs;
- to consider agreeing to audio-visual recordings being made of sessions, with the option of not being visible or audible on any recordings
- to agree to adhere to confidentiality recommendations;
- not to use any form of social media during the attendance of MFT sessions.

The section of the contract for the practitioners/institution can cover the following issues:

- to be on time for all scheduled sessions;
- to notify the group well in advance if not able to attend;
- to be respectful, non-violent and non-discriminatory to everyone attending MFT;
- not to attend MFT when under the influence of alcohol or drugs;
- to agree to preserve confidentiality of information except as required by law or in other limited circumstances (e.g., child protection issues, suicidal or homicidal intent, court order);
- to record meetings for supervision/training purposes – and respect the wishes of those group members who do not wish to be captured on video.

Inclusion and exclusion criteria

MFT works best when participating families have similar issues in common, such as the psychological or physical illness or disorder of one or more of its members, problems in school with a threat of the student being permanently excluded or various forms of intra-family violence. Having their child placed in a residential setting or in-patient unit is yet another 'common denominator' that some families will have in common. In other words, having a problem or issue in common is the main inclusion criteria for attending bespoke multi-family group work.

There are several exclusion criteria, some of which are general, whereas others are temporary. A general exclusion criterion applies to parents or other carers who have a conviction of child sexual abuse or where there is a risk or suspicion of ongoing or potential child sexual abuse. Adults and adolescents with a history of indiscriminate violence against strangers should not be included in MFT. Intra-family violence is not an exclusion criterion; however, a detailed risk assessment needs to precede the inclusion of such individuals in MFT.

Temporary exclusion criteria cover a number of situations, like when a group member is for a limited period of time not able to attend MFT, such as during an acute psychotic episode or due to a phase of alcohol or drug intoxication. The main reason for excluding individual group members at that point is to avoid potentially disruptive behaviours. The fact that an important family member (one of the parents or a symptomatic child or young person) is not attending MFT is *not* a reason the rest of the family cannot participate in MFT, and it is therefore not an exclusion criterion. What constitutes a 'family' has to be a very flexible notion and should be discussed but be left to members of the 'family' to define for themselves. Hence separated parents, step-parents, grandparents, uncles and aunts should all be welcomed to MFT; indeed, anyone who is part of the children's or adults' caring network should be. There are many families who, for a variety of reasons, are reluctant to attend MFT. Such reluctance is *not* an exclusion criterion, and an enforced treatment context has proved helpful, particularly with families presenting with severe child protection issues. In these cases, social care professionals may tell parents that MFT attendance is the only alternative to the removal of a child from their care.

Chapter 2

Does it work, and how can we make it work better?

The evidence base

The gathering of evidence about an intervention's efficacy and effectiveness is necessary to influence commissioners and policy makers. It is also important to provide service users who are considering engaging with an intervention information about the likely success of that intervention. However, evidence-based practice (and practice-based evidence) should not be seen solely as a means to an end. Practitioners have an ethical responsibility not just to use interventions that are supported by evidence but to continuously interrogate, evaluate and develop practice based on *both* research findings *and* feedback and observations from one's own clinical work.

There is a need for more rigorous research to understand both the effectiveness and mechanisms of change involved with MFT. Furthermore, it is hard to draw meaningful general conclusions from existing research due to the diversity of the theoretical models, interventions, settings, intensities and combination of MFT with other therapeutic interventions. Van Es et al. (2023) provide an overview of existing controlled trials focusing on the impact of MFT on mental health problems and family functioning. They identified a total of 31 peer-reviewed, controlled studies evaluating the effect of MFT and 16 trials which could be included in their meta-analysis. All but one of the studies were deemed at risk of bias, with problems concerning confounding variables, selection of participants and missing data. The authors were able to confirm that MFT is offered in diverse settings, with studies presenting a variety of therapeutic modalities, focal problems and populations. However, due to the large amount of heterogeneity, they were unable to draw meaningful general conclusions about efficacy by combining all the studies. While several individual studies report positive findings, including improvements in mental health, vocational outcomes and social functioning, the authors, nevertheless, concluded that more methodologically rigorous research is needed to further examine the potential benefits of MFT and its core components (van Es et al., 2023).

Gelin et al. (2018) provide an overview of the literature regarding MFT's applications to major psychiatric disorders and conclude that MFT's strongest evidence base is for schizophrenia and chronic psychoses. The specific effectiveness

DOI: 10.4324/9781003442424-2

of psychoeducational MFT on relapse rates has been shown in an early study (McFarlane et al., 1995a). After a 4-year follow-up, comparisons between MFT with psychoeducation and MFT without psychoeducation tended to yield similar improvements in relapse rates, suggesting it maybe the multifamily format, rather than its actual theoretical orientation, that best explains MFT's efficacy. In line with this hypothesis, a subsequent randomized controlled trial (RCT) comparing an MFT programme limited to providing information and support (i.e., without its full psychoeducational component) with single-family intervention found equal improvements in both treatment arms, suggesting that the social interactions taking place among families in MFT may in themselves be as beneficial as the psychoeducational component of single family interventions (Mueser et al., 2001). Gelin et al. (2018) point to a promising growing body of evidence regarding the effectiveness of MFT for mood disorders (particularly in children), eating disorders and alcohol-substance abuse but conclude that more controlled research is needed for these conditions. They describe how other disorders such as anxiety disorders, autism and attention deficit hyperactivity disorder have been studied in a more anecdotal fashion and require more rigorous investigations. Cook-Darzens et al. (2018) provide an overview of the empirical literature regarding MFT applications to *non-psychiatric* conditions and problems and find apparent benefits of MFT approaches for family management of several severe chronic medical illnesses as well as prevention of educational failure and exclusion. However, like van Es et al. (2023), both Gelin et al. (2018) and Cook-Darzens et al. (2018) point to limitations with regard to methodological quality. Gelin et al. (2018) recommend that future research efforts focus on the specific advantage of MFT over other active treatment modalities, the comparative efficacy of various MFT models for a given population and MFT's change processes.

Regarding the question of effective components, or the 'therapeutic ingredients' of MFT, a systematic review of 22 studies involving process research on psychoeducational family interventions for psychosis (Grácio et al., 2016) identified different combinations of active ingredients depending on the method of exploration (qualitative explorations of participants' opinions and outcome-related mediating variables; quantitative process-outcome studies). Despite this diversity, therapeutic alliance, support and sharing were highly emphasized by most studies, followed by education and relatives' reframing of the patient's symptoms and, to a lesser extent, coping skills training.

Three studies on psychiatric day patients and inpatients suffering from major depression analysed families' reports of helpful and unhelpful experiences of MFT using interpretive phenomenological analysis (IPA) (Hellemans et al., 2011), content analysis (Lemmens et al., 2003) and self-report questionnaires (Lemmens et al., 2009). Results revealed the prominence of therapeutic factors that reflected the unique structural and process aspects of MFT (rather than specific interventions or exercises), such as group cohesion and support and experiences of communality, as well as learning by observation of and identification with other families. Insight, hope and self-disclosure were also highly valued. Overall, a high level of satisfaction with MFT, both by therapists and families, is suggested by high rates of treatment adherence and of reported helpful experiences (Lemmens et al., 2003; Valdez et al., 2013). MFT programmes for eating disorders gathered information about families' experiences using IPA and other phenomenological methods (Engman-Bredvik & Suarez, 2016; Gelin et al., 2016), daily rating scales and journals, researcher observations and focus groups (Voriadaki et al., 2015) and content analysis of structured open-ended interviews. In addition to these factors, these studies reported improved understanding of the disorder, enhanced motivation for recovery for the adolescents, improved family dynamics and parental self-efficacy and increased ability to express emotions and movements of group affiliation and differentiation as change mechanisms. Several studies (for example, Morris et al., 2014; Hazel et al., 2004; McDonell et al., 2006; McFarlane, 2016; McFarlane et al., 1995b) also captured the benefits of MFT on the psychological and physical wellbeing of family members. This could be considered both a positive outcome *and* a mechanism of change, as improvement in the well-being of family members is likely to be associated with improvement for the 'identified patient'.

We do not yet know in what circumstances MFT is optimal as a stand-alone primary intervention because it is often administered in combination with other treatments and support. MFT often emerges as a valuable treatment option because of its cost effectiveness, but this assertion requires further exploration given that it is often offered alongside other interventions. There is a need for research to focus on the interaction between MFT and other treatments, its potential 'added value' and the groups for whom it is most likely to 'work'. For example, Pérez-García et al. (2020) conducted a randomized control trial comparing the efficacy of multifamily therapy with individual therapy as usual for adolescents attending an outpatient mental health centre in southeastern Spain. They found no significant differences in externalizing or internalizing symptoms between the two interventions at 6 months and 1 year of the intervention. However, the analysis of main factors indicated greater treatment as usual efficacy in the domain of externalizing behaviour, whereas MFT showed greater efficacy in internalizing behaviour. Eisler et al. (2016) conducted a multi-centre RCT of 167 families with adolescents experiencing anorexia nervosa receiving either single-family therapy or a combination of single-family therapy and MFT. The MFT group gained significantly more weight, and a greater number of MFT patients achieved a good or intermediate outcome (Eisler et al., 2016). Van Es et al. (2023) also highlight the need to understand the interaction between MFT and other treatment approaches; for example, individual trauma-focused treatment may be most effective to alleviate symptoms of PTSD, while MFT may be indicated to support family interactions that suffer the consequences of the disorder, whereas for patients with schizophrenia, it is more likely that psychoeducation offered to family members would be beneficial (van Es et al., 2023).

In order to progress the field of research exploring the effectiveness of MFT, there is a need for more rigorous research. Van Es et al. (2023) suggest that researchers should provide a clear explanation of the therapeutic modalities and techniques used and a description of how the program was adapted to suit the needs of the specific target group as well as using a structured manual and training facilitators to improve the implementation and replication of the program. After all, MFT covers a wide range of therapeutic modalities and therapeutic aims. Clinicians and researchers have suggested that MFT touches upon factors that other therapies cannot reach (Jewell & Lemmens, 2018; Schmidt & Asen, 2005), suggesting that the added value of MFT might be social support (McFarlane, 2016) or the interaction between participants from different families, including mutual feedback and support (Hellemans et al., 2011; Jewell & Lemmens, 2018; Lemmens et al., 2009). However, it has to be acknowledged that both the relative impact of MFT on mental health outcomes and the mechanisms of MFT that contribute towards any change require further investigation and evaluation.

Evaluating practice

The evidence base for MFT is more developed in some areas than others. However, a lack of evidence should not prevent the use of MFT to help families so long as: a) there is a clear rationale for doing so, b) it is not being offered in place of a treatment that would be likely to be more effective and c) there is an explicit commitment to learn from practice. In these situations, a cautious approach is recommended. In addition to a clear rationale as to why MFT is being offered, the practitioners should present a logic model (see Figure 2.1.) clearly describing *inputs* (what they are going to do), *outputs* (what they expect to change) and hypothesized *mechanisms of change* (how the change happens). In this way the practitioners are both holding themselves to account as well as creating a framework from which they can explicitly learn and develop their practice. Before trialling any intervention, the input of potential service users and other stakeholders is essential. By asking for their views, one can obtain important information about the viability of the intervention and the proposed ways of capturing change. For example, children who are not attending school may inform practitioners that they would be prepared to attend a family class (see Chapter 10) in school but *not* during school hours. Parents may similarly report that, due to work or childcare commitments, they would not be able to attend a family class during the school day. Parents may state that, from their perspective, the proposed outcome measures would not capture what is important to them or that there were too many or too long questionnaires to complete.

Where the existing evidence base is not strong for a MFT project, the intervention should first be trialled and evaluated on a small scale. Detailed feedback from both the outcome measures and interviews with families can be combined with the clinical observations of practitioners and used explicitly to inform any decisions about developing and expanding the intervention further. Where the evidence base is stronger, practice should still be evaluated against a logic model. If there is a good 'fit' between the evidence base and the proposed intervention, it can often be 'scaled up' more quickly. In these cases, the information gathered from the evaluation is more likely to serve the function of 'fine-tuning' the intervention and understanding whether and how it works in the specific service context.

Designing an outcomes framework

Practitioners using MFT generally share a wish to reach the families they want to help, to engage these families and to keep them engaged through the process. However, some desired outcomes will differ significantly between practitioners. For example, some might be looking to improve school attendance; others might be looking to reduce the chance a child has to be removed from their parent's care; others may hope to see young people sustain and gain weight and so on. Furthermore, desired outcomes and delivery context have a role in shaping an MFT project regarding where, how and how often it is delivered. However, despite the range of outcomes MFT practitioners aim for, and the variety of contexts where MFT is delivered, there are common *mechanisms of change*, the reasons *why* we think families improve across most MFT projects. These are listed in Box 3.

Box 3   Potential mechanisms of change in MFT

- Joining with families who experience similar difficulties reduces feelings of social isolation, stigmatization and shame. This is both therapeutic and creates a context where families are more open to learn and change.
- MFT activities expose families to new relational experiences and perspectives which strengthen reflectiveness and mentalization capacity in relation to their own actions and situations.
- Families discover and build on competencies and practice new skills, communications and behaviours in a safe space.
- Families are supported by other families and held accountable for change by thinking about how they can transfer what they have learnt to their 'real life' and report back to the group.
- Feelings of competence and solidarity are further improved by contributing to solutions to other people's difficulties.

Capturing desired outcomes

When designing an outcomes framework, it makes sense to clearly link outcome measures with desired 'outputs'. For example, a MFT project for children who are not attending school might look at attendance rates and engagement with learning, as well as factors that they hypothesize are linked to non-attendance, such as child emotional and behavioural functioning, engagement with school, parent–school relationships and parent–child relationships. To capture outcomes, it can be helpful to look at outcome studies in one's area of work and, if possible and appropriate, to use the same outcome measures. This allows some rudimentary comparison between the outcomes one is seeing and those found by others.

Many outcome measures are symptom based and, as such, closely aligned with a medical model of mental health and a bias in favour of white, western constructions of mental health. Including self-report measures of general well-being or the impact of problems on daily life in outcomes frameworks can make them less culturally biased, as can the inclusion of goal-based ratings. To improve equity further, measures should be translated into service users' primary language where appropriate. The cognitive and developmental level of the responder also needs to be carefully considered. Younger children can be asked to provide feedback via visual analogue scales, such as the Child Outcome Rating Scale (Casey et al., 2020) or play-based qualitative feedback. Individuals with lower levels of education or presenting with learning difficulties may need to be assisted to complete measures or provided with simplified measures. If there is scope, one can also examine potential mechanisms of change that are hypothesized to be associated with good outcomes. In the case of an MFT project to increase school attendance, for example, these might include an improvement in the 'match' between the child and the school setting or more effective mentalizing in the parent–child relationship.

It is important to consider the potential burden on families of completing outcome measures and to be aware that there is a difference between service evaluation and research. When families take part in research, they go through a process of giving informed consent, which means that they must understand what will be required of them; they need to understand why data are being collected, and they are required to formally agree to take part. They also need to agree that data obtained from research projects can be more widely disseminated to inform work in the field. Furthermore, the process that families go through as part of a research project must be approved by an independent ethics committee. By contrast, in the case of a service evaluation, consent is obtained locally to gather data with a view to service improvement but by giving consent, families are *not* agreeing to take part in a research study, and there is no independent ethical oversight. The burden on families in terms of data collection should reflect this by being minimal and clearly relevant to service improvement. It should be made clear to all families contributing to service evaluation or research that their participation is entirely voluntary and will not impact the service they receive (see www.hra-decisiontools.org.uk/research/for guidance on differentiating research, audit and evaluation). Finally, it is important to acknowledge that the very process of administering questionnaires can have an impact on family members' responses, particularly if measures are administered by the practitioner. For example, a parent might not feel free to express their true views about a project or may underreport their difficulties because they do not want to offend the practitioner or because of the power differential they experience in relation to that practitioner. For this reason alone, it is, if possible, useful to have an independent person to administer the measures and conduct feedback interviews. Families can also be asked to provide feedback via apps or online forms.

Making sense of outcome data

There are many covariate factors both at baseline and over the course of treatment that might influence outcomes. Baseline factors including social, cultural and contextual/familial factors as well as the severity and chronicity of difficulties may differentiate who responds (or how strongly they respond) to MFT. For example, it might be hypothesized that children from minority ethnic groups respond more strongly to MFT than CBT because the model uses families' own ideas of illness and recovery rather than imposing a westernized construction of mental health. Similarly, intervening factors that take place during the course of treatment (such as significant life events) can also affect outcomes. In many cases MFT is not used as a 'stand-alone' intervention, and other inputs may be offered alongside it either prior to or during the course of a group. Where this is the case, the relative impact of such interventions on outcomes and any potential interaction between MFT and the (other) intervention is important to understand. For example, it might be hypothesized that children from minority ethnic groups who receive *both* MFT and CBT do better than those who receive CBT alone because they develop coping strategies that help with their symptomology, *and* their families are able to be engaged in their recovery in a way that is more culturally reflexive. Finally, outcomes can vary as a result of differences in staff skill level and service delivery context. It is not possible in small-scale evaluation projects to investigate the impact of covariate factors in any depth, but it is important to be curious about these from the outset. Practitioners can use existing research to help them identify potential covariate factors and bear them in mind when interpreting outcomes, making clinical decisions and planning future research. Small-scale service evaluation data are usually not sufficiently robust to make generalizable assertions but can be a helpful guide for decision making, especially when interpreted alongside existing research findings, and they can also provide a foundation for larger-scale, more rigorous research.

Gathering qualitative data

The collation of qualitative data allows one to move beyond the question of 'does it work?' towards 'why does it work or not work?' and 'how can we make it work better?' There are various ways to ask families about their experiences of MFT. If their views are being included as part of an ethically approved research project, there is the opportunity to conduct in-depth interviews and analysis and focus on specific issues of interest. Where this is not possible because of resource or service setting constraints, a 'lighter touch' approach can be taken. Families can be invited to meet, speak on the phone or complete a survey remotely. To provide some brief feedback, families can be asked what they liked about MFT, what they didn't like, what they found helpful, what they would change and so on. It can be helpful to add a question about whether they felt MFT was respectful of their culture. People from minoritized backgrounds may not feel comfortable bringing this up spontaneously themselves but may be more likely to share their views if directly asked.

Information gained via qualitative data can provide important insight that enriches one's understanding of an intervention beyond outcome measures. For example, an outcome measure may tell one that a child is less anxious and is attending school more regularly, but interviews with families can provide more nuanced information that helps one understand why these changes have happened. Qualitative information can also provide information that is missed by outcome measures. For example, one may hear reports from parents and children that the reason that school attendance has improved was because the child had made more friends, a finding perhaps not picked up by the outcome measures used. As a result of obtaining this information, one may decide to include some measure of social functioning with outcomes that are co-produced with the child and focus a little more on the issue of friendships in MFT sessions. Finally, qualitative data can be important in identifying important contextual factors that may be acting as moderators. For example, through interviews with parents and children it may emerge that a small number of parents from minority ethnic groups found it harder to make connections with the rest of the families who were from perceived ethnic majority groups. Ethnicity therefore could emerge as a potential moderating factor and provide a focus for future interventions. This example also shows how differences in outcomes and experiences that can be missed by outcome measures can be captured by qualitative evaluation. Finally, asking families directly for their views on how an intervention can be developed gives them the agency that they are entitled to in their unique and valuable position as the recipients of the intervention: a privileged position that practitioners do not hold.

Pulling it together: Example of a logic model

One way of summarizing an evaluation framework is via a logic model (see Figure 2.1). A simplified hypothetical logic model for a multi-family group to support children not attending school is presented in the following. A logic model is a short-hand way of communicating *what* practitioners intend to do, *why* they intend to do it, *how* they think it will work and *which* outcomes they expect to emerge as a result. Factors that are likely to moderate outcomes are also identified.

The process of developing a logic model can often enable fine-tuning of an intervention. For example, the intervention could be refined on the basis of feedback from teachers and children. Initially a multi-family group like this may be targeted at any student whose attendance is below 30%. However, if teachers and families fed back that there were specific issues faced by children with a neurodevelopmental diagnosis, such as ASD or ADHD, that were not common to the whole group, the intervention could be tailored accordingly. Similarly, if children aged under 14 reported that they would not be comfortable in a group with older children, a decision might be made to run separate groups for children aged 11–14 and those aged 14 and older. In addition to academic research, more general sources of

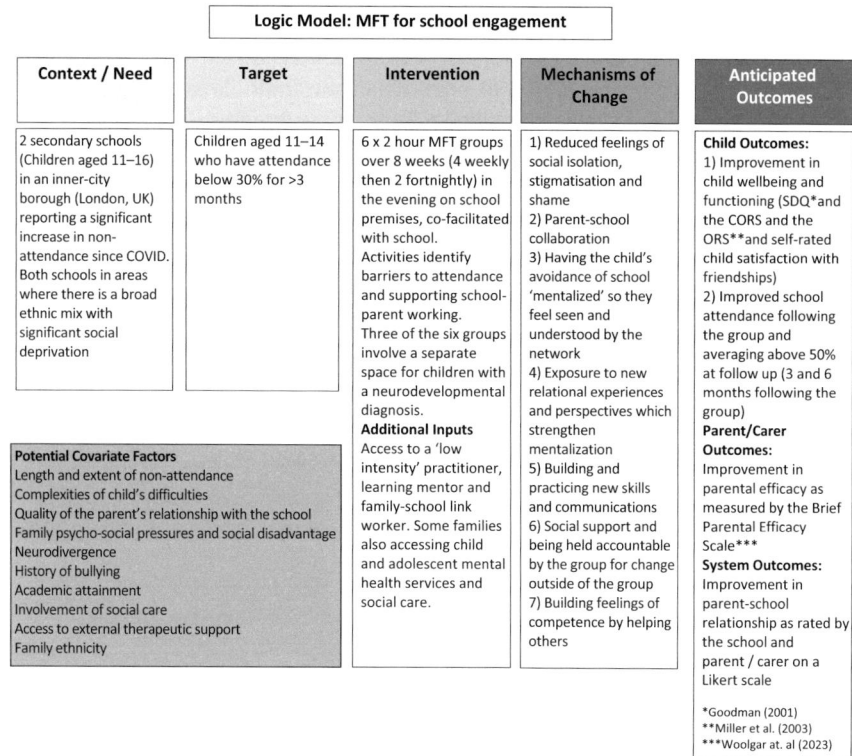

Figure 2.1 Logic model to support service evaluation of an MFT group for school engagement

information can be used to inform logic models, such as reports and findings from special interest groups and learning from local or similar services, other organizations and other practitioners.

Learning from evaluation

A framework for evaluation is only the first step when developing MFT projects. Once data have been collated, the logic model can be refined, interventions developed and, where appropriate, findings more widely disseminated to inform the work of other practitioners. With small numbers it is not possible to perform meaningful statistical analysis or make generalizable claims, though single case studies and in-depth qualitative studies can yield rich data. If families have successfully engaged in MFT and measures indicate positive outcomes, a decision may be made to extend the intervention. However, to fulfil the ethical responsibility to continuously examine and develop one's clinical practice and to involve service users in this process, evaluation findings need to be considered. With an outcomes framework in place over a period of time, data from multiple groups and, potentially, multiple settings can be combined to more robustly improve both our understanding and practice of MFT intervention and used as a basis for larger-scale, more robust research studies.

Chapter 3

Basic techniques

The formation of sub-groups and other context changes

Even though MFT is a group approach, this does not mean that all families always need to be together in a large group which is composed of all participants. It is, in fact, desirable to form a variety of sub-groups, requiring families and their members, as well as the practitioners, to negotiate several context shifts within a short space of time. We have already emphasized the need for practitioners to be active, flexible and multi-positional. When this stance is visible to families, it can become 'catching' as they themselves get better at managing context shifts. Each sub-group, or mini-context, requires participants to adopt different roles and positions, and the work with the large group can be intensified by creating sub-groups from time to time. This can take place in different constellations. One can form sub-groups of two or three families or have a group of children and a group of parents work at the same time in different rooms or in different spaces in the same room. It can also be useful for groups of fathers, mothers, children or siblings to work separately on certain topics. Subgroups tend to work more intensively and focused, particularly when the discussion in the large group beforehand has been slow or lacking. The subsequent exchange of thoughts and experiences between the members of subgroups is then often surprisingly lively and allows group members to share their ideas and experiences. Practitioners can also use this technique to activate all the members of a lethargic large group, which can be quite strenuous.

MFT demands that family members move in and out of multiple roles, from 'patient' to 'expert', from 'victim' to 'witness', from 'helpless' to 'agentive'. It is learning through doing rather than by just talking and listening. Taking on changing positions encourages group participants to change their perspectives, either by talking directly to other individuals or families about a particular issue, speaking up in the large group or just relating in different ways in ad-hoc mini-contexts. Sub-groups can also be formed according to gender, age and other characteristics, such as mothers meeting just with mothers in a 30 minutes while fathers talk during this time to other fathers and children spend time with other children. These

DOI: 10.4324/9781003442424-3

three sub-groups would meet in parallel, and their ideas and suggestions can be fed back to the large group subsequently. It is important to note that meeting in a large circle is only *one* of the many contexts utilized in MFT, and it is not necessarily the most conducive one when it comes to exchanging thoughts and feelings, as it is very likely that some group participants are too shy to contribute with so many other people listening. Yet there are others who simply love dominating the conversation in front of a large audience. Unlike in traditional group therapy where the work always involves *all* the participants being together, MFT promotes work in sub-groups and sometimes even work with a single family or couple or just one individual.

It may be worth emphasizing once again that MFT practitioners need not only be flexible with their eyes and bodies but also flexible in their conceptual positions and how these need to change. In the first few groups, they usually need to be rather central and directive, as at this point the responsibility for the therapeutic context may rest solely with them: they are the 'context makers'. It is their job to sense the 'group mood' and create a setting with a comfortable 'climate' to enable group members to open up and share their experiences and reflections. As the group develops cohesion and purpose, the practitioners will begin to de-centralize themselves, only to step forward again if required in response to the group entering new territory, when having to manage a specific challenge or when group dynamics are becoming unstable. Even in these situations, the practitioners will have to make a careful assessment and create a new context that minimizes their involvement and maximizes the families' resources.

Practitioners are continuously considering how they can create contexts that de-centralize themselves over the course of a group but also throughout each session, and this can involve positioning themselves repeatedly in different ways. The metaphor of an eagle who flies high and circles 'prey' may describe one particular position practitioners can assume: from a bird's-eye perspective, it is possible to spot problematic intra- or inter-family interactions and intervene. The practitioners can then decide to 'fly in', as it were, and change into a 'benign' woodpecker, focusing on and highlighting a particular issue or interaction. Having done so, usually for only brief moments and certainly no longer than 1 minute, the practitioner can then again return to the 'circling' observer position until the next opportunity for potential intervention is spotted. An example may explain this process more clearly: An activity like the Family Website requires all families to work in parallel on a task, with the practitioners standing back and observing intra-family interactions from a meta perspective. During this activity the practitioners notice that one particular family is struggling to engage a reluctant child, with the parents becoming increasingly frustrated. The practitioners may decide to 'fly in', apply the five-step model (see below), get family members to respond and then quickly withdraw back to an observer position, circling again like an eagle, as it were, and being on the lookout for problematic interactions occurring in other families.

Making and re-making contexts for change

How, then, do practitioners make decisions on how and when to intervene and how to make and re-make larger and smaller working contexts? A clinical example may help to illustrate this. Let us imagine that in the large group planning meeting at the beginning of an MFT session, several group members identify the theme of 'managing and controlling hyperactive children' and feel that this should be a major focus of MFT that day. This should pose the following question for the MFT practitioners: 'what are the contexts that we need to create to address the presenting problem?' When answering this basic question pragmatically, it is helpful to consider four context dimensions: *person*, *time*, *activity* and *place* (Asen, 2004).

The Person Context relates to *who* should be involved in a meeting or activity addressing the issue of hyperactive children: should it be whole families? Or should it be three separate groups composed of parents only or mothers only and fathers only, and what about working with children only? Or should children not be involved? Should one involve members of the parents'/partners' support network? What about high-conflict families post-separation: should ex-partners be included in MFT or not? In other words, there is a considerable choice of scenarios involving different members of the group and beyond.

The next consideration is the Time Context: *when* to address the hyperactivity issue. This can be defined in terms of the actual time: should it be addressed immediately or at a later stage? If it is addressed, how many minutes or hours will be spent on it? The MFT practitioners will need to consider the pros and cons of various options.

How to address the issue brings us to the third context dimension, which we have termed the Activity Context. This context includes, of course, therapeutic conversations or discussions that tend to be word focused. However, MFT uses many playful activities, some of which are nonverbal or paraverbal, such as role plays, sculpting, collages, games and various exercises. The therapeutic activities are fitted to the presenting issues and may change from session to session, and Chapter 6 describes many of these activities.

The Place Context – the *where* – is the fourth context dimension. MFT is usually carried out in one or two large rooms located in a health service or social care setting or in a school. But MFT can also take place in the street, in shopping centres and markets or even on public transport (buses, trams, trains, boats), depending on the issues one wants to address. With hyperactive children, for example, a public or shopping centre may make it more likely that one can study reported problems 'in vivo' and, with the help of other families, invite experimentation with new coping strategies.

It is important to emphasize that the contextualizing questions *who? when? what?* and *where?* need to be asked not only at the beginning of taking on new work but throughout the whole process of conducting MFT. By increasingly involving individuals and families in this questioning process, it becomes possible to co-construct relevant contexts for change, thereby opening up new ways of seeing and experiencing. It is important that practitioners, together with family members, try to review continuously whether the established *who, when, what* and *where* contexts are still helpful.

Playing the 'Systemic Quartet'

One way of conceptualizing systemic MFT work is to think about it having four distinct phases, which could be described by using a musical metaphor, the Systemic Quartet. String quartets, one of the highlights of classical music, involve four instrumentalists playing chamber music. Most string quartets consist also of four 'movements', similar to the sequential 'moves' of MFT. The first 'move', like the first movement of a string quartet, which is often an 'allegro', consists of identifying a theme. This is done collaboratively with group members and the practitioners who identify and focus on a seemingly problematic relationship or communication pattern. This is followed by the second 'movement', in string quartet music often a 'scherzo', which invites experimentation so that hopefully non-problematic interactions and communications can emerge, and this is often achieved with the help of MFT activities (see Chapter 6). The practitioners' third 'move' or 'movement', in music often a thoughtful contemplative 'andante', involves reflecting on what has been experienced during the second movement. The last therapeutic phase, the fourth 'movement', the 'finale', aims to initiate a transfer of what has been experienced and learned in the session to everyday life outside the group, be that the home, school or work. It is here that homework tasks which families carry out between sessions can have a place. The four main ingredients of the therapeutic process can be succinctly described as follows: *identifying, experimenting, reflecting* and *transferring.*

In practical steps, a MFT session can be started with *identifying* a theme and/or preoccupation which most group participants have in common. This is often done by asking the families themselves, but in specific projects (see Chapters 8, 9 and 10) the majority of themes may be pre-determined and based on qualitative research and experience other practitioners have passed on. In the previous example, the theme is 'controlling hyperactive children'. The *experimenting* move consists of an activity in which all families and their members participate, like in the Remote Control activity, which usually elicits plenty of both surprise and laughter. In the subsequent *reflecting* phase, group members consider and exchange their ideas and experiences, with the help of mentalizing techniques (see Chapter 4). However, the work is not completed, as the *transferring* move(ment) has to be 'played' first to consider how any new ways of thinking and doing experienced in the group can be exported home. This is best done by creating a homework task, like, in this case example, each family constructing a remote control for use at home with the most important buttons.

The five-step intervention model

MFT practitioners work 'live' in the 'here and now', observing and naming inter-family as well as intra-family processes. They actively search for 'live' examples of potentially problematic interactions. As soon as these appear, the practitioners can pause and become benignly curious about what is going on in a family or group members. *The five-step intervention model* (Asen, 1997) is a basic systemic intervention technique which consists of five separate, though linked, steps that practitioners can take in order to address and/or intervene in specific interactions and communications they have observed.

The *first step* consists of a plain observational statement about a potentially problematic interaction the practitioners have identified. This is prefaced by a sentence like 'I notice that . . '. or 'I have observed that . . . . '. The following are a few examples:

I notice that . . .

- *you, Mum, want Emma to put her coat on, but she does not do this . . . .*
- *you, Jack, have decided to do exactly the opposite of what your Mum is telling you . . .*
- *you parents want to talk to each other, but Philip continually interrupts you . . .*
- *whenever Dad begins to say something, Mum intervenes and completes his sentence . . .*
- *you stand back while others do the work as if that's the best way to help them . . .*
- *your daughter seems to like Harriet's father a lot; she hardly knows him but sits on his lap and cuddles up to him . . .*

The *second step* consists of the practitioners checking their observation with others. This is not only with persons directly but also with the whole group or members from other families: '*Do you, or does anyone else here, also see it that way, or am I totally off the mark?*' Putting it like this emphasizes that what is being said is merely a subjective observation and signals that practitioners are aware that they can simply not know in advance whether their observations are shared by others and therefore need to check them. If group members do not know what the practitioner is talking about, then it is best not to insist on the accuracy or sheer brilliance of the voiced observations but to retract them by stating: '*We probably got that wrong'*. This also exemplifies the stance of humility and the not-knowing position, both important principles of systemic work.

However, if the people generally agree with the observational statement, it is time for the *third step*, to invite evaluation from the concerned individual, family or group members or indeed the larger group: '*Are you happy that it is this way, or do you mind?*' This question is meant to be open ended and allows each person to reply with 'yes' or 'no' and should then lead them to explain how they arrived at their respective positions. The practitioners can explore in detail why specific answers have been given and how they connect up, if at all. Mostly the response will be that other people share the observations, and this allows moving to steps four and five. However, if the general answer is a whole-hearted 'no' and the practitioners still insist on pursuing the same line of inquiry, then they are likely to meet a lot of resistance. For example, if parents say that they do not mind that their child continues to scream, the practitioners can observe: '*You say that you don't mind that Jack continues to scream; what might be the advantages and disadvantages of that? What do other families here think?*' At times this helps parents or other group members to identify what is appropriate and what is not and what the implications of challenging a child or a parent are. The aim is always for practitioners and group members to work together, and if a family or some of its members does not agree with the observations of the practitioners, the latter need to accept and not get caught up in a symmetrical escalation but stimulate reflective thinking instead by, for example, stating: '*You say that you do not mind if Jack continues screaming, and from what you have told us, he screams day and night at home and in the nursery. What do you think are the advantages and disadvantages if he continues to scream here for another few hours? What would happen in the nursery? What might be the consequences? What do other families here think?*' In this way, group members, young and old, are invited to consider the pros and cons of action or inaction.

The *fourth step* encourages group member(s) to give voice to their views about change: '*So, if you do not want things to continue in this way, how would you like it to be?*' In this example, a parent may reply: '*Well, that's obvious, we want him to stop screaming!*' The practitioners follow this up by taking the *fifth step* to get the parent or child to identify how to go about achieving this change: '*What would you have to say or do now to make it be the way you want it to be? What would be the first step?*'

This seemingly concrete and simple format for framing and intervening helps practitioners to pinpoint and address emerging interactions in the 'here and now'. Often families behave as if they have no ideas about what to do differently, and they almost inevitably turn to the practitioners' guidance and advice. They see them as 'experts' and view and present themselves as 'helpless'. However, instead of merely answering questions put to them by families in a straightforward manner, practitioners can refer to the expertise of other group members, for example, by asking: '*What is stopping you from doing what you think you should be doing? What is the first little thing you might need to do? Who else here has some ideas? Mrs Wood, what do you think about the question Mr Jones asked? How would you answer it?*' These questions are designed to activate and involve other group members, and once there have been responses, the practitioners can continue: '*Who here would like to say something about the issues raised by Mrs Wood? Are these issues that might also be familiar to others in the room here?*' The practitioners may also focus on another observed specific interaction, like between a child, Jack, and his parents: '*What would you say about what you observed going on between Jack and his parents? I noticed that Jack always blames his parents for getting things wrong – is there anyone else here who has noticed this, or am I just imagining this?*'

If you were to find yourselves in a situation like this, what might you want to do, how about you over there?' These and similar questions aim to draw in, bit by bit, the expertise of other group members and invite them to offer their own perspectives and ideas.

Interviewing techniques

In the initial phase of MFT, the practitioners' main aim is to engage families and help them to connect with each other and share problems. This requires practitioners to be rather central, trying to explain principles, shaping the agenda and reassuring group members that it is safe to talk not only to them but above all to other families and their members. To achieve this, practitioners need to use containing language, being accepting and non-challenging. However, in gradually moving to no longer giving answers or advice, the practitioners can make use of *circular and reflexive questioning* (Selvini Palazzoli et al., 1980), an elegant technique which was developed for single-family therapy but can be used equally well in MFT. It enables practitioners to move away from being 'experts' to a position of becoming 'curious inquirers' who solicit information about people's beliefs and perceptions regarding relationships. By responding to the feedback provided, the practitioner enacts 'circularity', basing the next question on the previous answer. Reflexive and circular questions can be asked with just one person present as well as when several families are present. Eliciting such information in their presence and asking them to comment and reflect on the answers given by the various individuals creates an infinite set of feedback loops which themselves change the fabric of family and group interactions. Each person could be asked the same question in turn, noting, if not commenting on, the different answers elicited. Triadic questions are particularly useful in that each person is asked to comment on the thoughts, behaviours and relationships of other group or family members. Engaged in such conversations, they also have the opportunity to be observers of others' perceptions about themselves rather than being involved in the action. Examples of different types of circular and reflexive questions (adapted from Selvini Palazzoli et al., 1980; Tomm, 1988) are contained in Box 4.

Box 4   Types of circular and reflexive questions

1. **Problem questions** *(these aim to define the history of the problem, the contexts within which it occurs and the differing responses to it)*

   - Who first noticed your problem? Who second? Who last? Who is most distressed?
   - What is your explanation for the problem?

- What is your partner's/father's/mother's explanation as to why you are having this problem? Do you agree with their view?
- What do you think made them form this opinion?
- If you wanted to change their mind about their view of your problem, how would you go about it?
- When the problem occurs, who does what in response to the problem?
- How does the problem affect spouse/father/mother/children?
- When you're depressed/have pain, who responds to it first. . . . What does s/he say or do? What happens next? How do you respond to his/ her response? What happens then? And what is your response to that?
- Is there anybody who thinks that your problem is not 'real'? Or someone who believes that you are not ill but just awkward? What is your response to that? What type of conversations between you and X does that produce?
- How come that X has this opinion? Do you think that X thinks that you could act differently? How do you know this? How good are you at working out what X or Y really thinks about your problem?
- What else might X or Y think or feel that they do not let you know about? How might they talk about your problem in your absence?
- What would you have to do to find out?
- If you did, what sort of responses might you get?
- I notice that Bill somehow manages to give his parents a lecture on how to listen to him. Which of the other families has noticed that? Who wants to say something about that?
- Who here wants to comment on what's going on between Jackie and her parents?

2. **Help questions** *(these aim to clarify who wants help for what, as well as the implications of seeking and receiving help)*

- Who in your family wants help most/who wants it least? What is your explanation for these differences?
- Who of the other people in the room have been in that situation? If you were in that position, what might you have done or do?
- How did you decide that you should come and get some help? How did you discuss this and with whom? What were the sort of responses?
- What would have happened if you had decided not to come to MFT?
- Does coming here for help make it easier or more difficult to discuss these things with your partner, friends, extended family?
- Supposing you weren't coming here for help, how would you deal with this problem?
- What does your mother/father/partner really think about you coming here for help? What do you think they imagine goes on here?

- Who'd be most/least in favour of you coping on your own rather than going for help?
- What do you think are the consequences if nothing is found which will help the problem? What will be the effects on you, on your partner/parent/child?

3. **Change questions** *(these aim to explore the implications and consequences of change)*

   - I am going to ask you a question to which the answer is probably very obvious: How would you know you're getting better? What sort of observations would you make? What would be different?
   - How would anybody else know?
   - Supposing you did not tell anybody that your problem had got better, would they notice anyway? What other signs would they observe that might make them think that you were getting better?
   - How would your partner/mother/child notice that you were getting better?
   - How would your relationship with your partner/mother be affected if your problem got better? What would be the advantages? Any disadvantages in getting better?
   - Supposing there were some disadvantages, and you decided that there might be something in it to keep the problems – would you be able to consciously produce them? What would you have to do? How would you go about doing this?
   - What would your partner's/mother's/father's response be if they knew?
   - Supposing there was no change in your problems for another few months – which relationship would suffer most?
   - Who here of the other families would like to say something about what you have just heard? Are these problems that others in the room are aware of as well?
   - You all heard the question Ms Sunshine asked me. What do you think of it? And how would you answer it?

4. **Relationship questions** *(these aim to examine communication and interaction patterns)*

   - How do you see the relationship between your brother and your mother? How do you think your father sees his relationship with you? How would your mother describe the relationship between you and your father? Would this be different from how you see it – or how your father sees it?
   - Who else in the group wants to answer these questions?
   - How do you explain the differences between how your father and your mother see this relationship?

- If your wife was sitting here and heard you say this, what might she say? And if she did say this, how would you respond? And what would be her reply?
- Who else here in the group has experienced something like that?
- Who is the closest/most distant to your father/mother? Who is second/ third most?
- Who agrees with you that X is closest to Y? Is there anyone who might have a different view? What do you think that is based on?
- Was there ever any time when this was different?
- What were things like before and after illness (death, separation) struck?
- When do you feel most like a daughter, when like a mother, when like a wife? How do you explain this? Who else can make you feel like that?
- Who is most/least upset when you do not get on with him/her/them?

5. **Hypothetical Questions** *(these aim to reflect on the implications of new scenarios and hypothetical situations)*

- If you weren't around . . . how would your parents get along without you?
- If one child would never leave home – who would it be?
- If you had not been born, what would your parents' marriage be like?
- If your wife got suddenly better, who would next be ill?
- If your wife spoke now, what might she say? And how might your father respond to that? And how would you respond to that?
- You have already got considerable experience with therapists and therapies. What would we have to do to make this therapy a failure too?
- Supposing your partner had been a fly on the wall throughout all our meetings . . . what would she think about it all? Would you agree with her observations? Why not?
- Supposing you let your husband negotiate all the contact with your mother and he took the responsibility for that . . . how would that affect your problems?
- If your mother were still alive today, what do you think her opinion would be about the problems you are having with the children?

Since attention in MFT groups can quickly wane among participants who are not directly involved in the interaction, circular questions are therefore not always followed and even understood by everyone. Active listening, a technique used in non-directive psychotherapy, can be very helpful in such a scenario: the practitioners try to repeat what has been said in their words *(lower level of active listening)*, to clarify content-related statements that were not made clear or to describe emotional backgrounds that were not addressed but could be hidden in the statement *(intermediate level of active listening)*. This signals to the individual, family or group that the practitioners are trying to understand them. At the same time, group members are given the opportunity to correct, expand or differentiate the statements. In a second step, the practitioners can repeat what a group member has said but now address it directly to the group or to another person. There are situations when practitioners start asking questions directly to one group member and find themselves quickly in one-to-one conversations, thereby potentially preventing interactions between group members. By using the *prompter technique*, the practitioners remain on the sidelines of the group and address a member of the group in the form of an aside that is sufficiently audible for other people: '*Lucy, do you want to know why John says he doesn't mind if his mother wakes him up in the morning? Does it intrigue you that his father doesn't say anything?*' or '*Mark, I can see you thinking while the group is chatting. Have you ever found yourself in the situation they're talking about? Yes? How did you feel then? It's interesting, you should tell them about it*'. The practitioners then withdraw, leaving it to other group members to continue the conversation.

Lieutenant Columbo's interviewing technique

Lieutenant Columbo, portrayed by the actor Peter Falk in the long-running American TV series, is a crime investigator who acts in a seemingly naïve, if not 'stupid', but benign and well-intentioned way. He embodies the 'not knowing position' and the stance of 'safe uncertainty' (Mason, 2019). Lieutenant Columbo appears to be slow and keeps sharing his hunches and observations with everyone as he goes along, displaying good intent as well as puzzlement. He often engages the people he wishes to interview in non-problem-oriented talk, getting into seemingly irrelevant detail, before closing in and nailing the chief suspect. Many of the phrases he employ can be put to good use by MFT practitioners (see Box 5).

Box 5 Lieutenant Columbo's words

'*Can I just check this?*'
'*When I was a kid, we had . . . .*'
'*That's funny . . . don't you have that . . . well, that's quite something . . .*'
'*Do you mind if I look around?*'
'*You don't happen to have a skeleton in the cupboard?*'
'*I think I am on a wild goose chase; can you help me?*'
'*I want to apologize for taking up your time . . .*'

'*Oh, one thing I almost forgot . . '.*
'*Oh, there I just one more thing . . .*'
'*To you, does it sound like a reasonable explanation?*'
'*I don't you want to get offended what I am going to say, but is it possible that you may have got that wrong?*'
'*There is a couple of loose ends I need to tie up . . .*'
'*Whatever happened to . . . .?*'
'*Makes you kind of wonder . . . it could be that, or it could be something else?*'
'*I know this sounds ridiculous, but it occurs to me that . . '.*
'*There is something I wanted to talk to you about . . '.*
'*I find it hard to believe, but . . '.*
'*Can you help me out with a problem I have . . .*'
'*I've got this hunch, but I may be wrong . . .*'

Structuring reflection time

Reflecting is the third 'movement' of the 'systemic quartet', and many of the previous questions lend themselves to inducing reflections during and after one of the many MFT activities. But how can one start the process? There are essentially two different ways of doing so. The first requires the practitioners to remain rather peripheral, merely activating everyone and setting short time limits: '*Can you think about what happened and what you experienced and talk about it for 2 minutes?*' The instruction can be vague like this or focused on a specific topic the practitioners name. They can then suggest different 'person contexts' with whom the talking and reflecting takes place: in pairs *('talk to your neighbour')*, in peer groups *('can all the fathers, all the mothers and all the young people form groups and think about this')*, in small groups which are randomly convened, in 'cross fostering' configurations (see subsequently) or via a slow *speed-dating* activity.

The second way of jump-starting reflecting processes is for the practitioners to take a more central position, focusing attention deliberately on a specific topic and initially leading the discussion, encouraging group members to engage to contribute. The large group can be split into two, with each practitioner leading one. Families or their members are invited to contribute to the discussion. The practitioners can focus on one family and demonstrate how to have a reflective discussion and then hand over to the members of this (now) 'expert' family to take over the practitioner's 'jobs' and to do the same with another family and for this to then be copied by all the other families.

It can be difficult to develop relevant questions that encourage families to reflect on both the MFT activity and its implications for their everyday lives. Questions cannot be merely limited to '*How did you feel?*' or '*How did it go for you?*', but resorting to the three-question technique can help here: the first question should be related to the experiential activity that just took place. The third question should be related to the actual problems and issues that people encounter on a daily basis and that was thematized during the experiential activity. The second question should link the two. For example, at the end of the Lie Detector activity, families could be asked the following three questions: '*How did you manage to discover the lie and the truths of the person you were talking to? What are the advantages and disadvantages of having lies detected? What would it be like if you started to guess more of each other's truths after you leave here today?*'

Reflecting teams

A considerable number of practices used in MFT are inspired by the 'reflecting team' concept (Andersen, 1987), based on the notion that an outside observer, be that an individual or a team, sees and experiences things differently from those who are directly involved in the therapeutic process. In MFT it is not only practitioners who have the potential for being a reflecting team but also the other families and their members. The *fishbowl technique* uses an inner and an outer circle. For example, teenagers (the 'fish') can in the inner circle discuss a specific theme among one another, with the parents (the 'cats') listening and observing this discussion. After some time, the positions are switched, with the parents then sitting in the inner circle, reflecting on the discussion they listened to and the teenagers now assuming the outer circle 'listening and observing' position. At a later stage the young people can return to the inner circle, reflecting on the reflections of their parents about their discussion. It is also possible, for example, to get mothers to discuss a particular issue and for the fathers to be in an observing position and then to switch over. The fishbowl scenario furthers inter-family interactions and makes people aware of the frequent circularity of these. This is a dedicated time slot for no longer than 10 minutes, during which action is temporarily suspended and time for reflection created, shifting from the heat of action to the relative coolness of contemplation. The practitioners may say: '*It's getting pretty hot here, a lot of noise, a lot of conflict. I think we should have a brief pause right away, to sit down and think about what's been happening just now*'. This can be a reflective 'taking the temperature' when all action is frozen for a brief time for everyone.

The 'outsider witness group' (White, 1995) is a ritualized technique that requires different group members provide their own personal responses and resonances as a form of feedback to a specific family or group dilemma or charged situation. It can be used, for example, when doing sculpting activities like Frozen Conflicts. When such sculpting takes place in the centre of the room, group members are invited to resonate with their personal views and feelings. Transfixed in their respective poses, it can be a powerful experience for members of the sculpted family to listen silently to how other families see them.

When engaging in multi-family work in day units (Asen & Scholz, 2010), it is also possible for practitioners to come together towards the end of one specific day each week, in a room away from the families, and to video-record their own reflections on, for example, how each family has managed a particular task or activity that day. The families can subsequently, in a 'fishbowl' setting, watch the video and offer their own reflections on the practitioners' reflections, with the practitioners being in a mere listening position.

Externalizing interventions

The practice of externalizing problem behaviours (White & Epston, 1990) aims to objectify problems instead of objectifying people. In other words, it is not the symptomatic person who is 'the problem', but the problem is separate from the person. These techniques aim to separate cognitions and behaviours linked with a problem or specific disorder from the personality of the individual, be that a child or adult. This allows family and group members joining forces against 'the illness' or 'the problem' rather than victimizing the problem bearer. The problem can be the illness or disorder (e.g., anorexia nervosa) or a symptom (e.g., hyperactivity in ADHD). The 'problem' can also be one of the following: a) abnormal cognitive patterns (e.g., the binge-purge-cycle in bulimia nervosa or the sudden emotional arousal one often sees with conduct disorders), b) relational patterns (e.g., the transgenerational cycles of high conflict) or c) developmental goals (e.g., the pathological dependencies in families with a chronically ill member). We are also mindful that a significant group of people do object to their 'diagnosis' (e.g., ASD or ADHD) being regarded as 'the problem' and that it is their view that being neurodivergent in a neurotypical world is 'the problem'.

Several externalizing activities are described in Chapter 6, for example, Wigglemon or Problem Portrait. These allow people to join forces against 'the illness' or 'the problem' rather than victimizing the problem bearer. As an example, a 'naughty child' does not retain this identity and is not equated with the problem, but the 'naughty behaviour' is decoupled from them and transported 'outside', being 'externalized' as, for example, 'red mist' which tends to haunt the child from time to time but which the child can slowly and gradually get to grips with through the help of the parents and significant others. The practitioners use more than just a technique when leading a discussion as follows: '*Is it possible that ADHD feels at home in this family? Has ADHD realized that it needs to make Dad angry at Teddy to drive a wedge between them and continue to rule?*' or '*Have you told your mother what Anorexia has in store for you in terms of reprisals if you're happy to eat?*'

Role reversals

Role reversals have much therapeutic potential, as participants assume an unfamiliar role within their own family. For example, children can be asked to act, for a limited time, as if they were their own parents – while the parents role play their children. The practitioners might introduce this activity in the following way: '*For the next 10 minutes, can each parent role play their child and each child their mother or father? Dear parents, in the role of your child you can be as well or badly behaved as you like, and you, dear children, as your own mum or dad try to take control over your children and try to manage them'.* The ensuing, hopefully benign, chaos is not only fun for all concerned but also rather informative: parents often report how surprised they were to hear their children, when role-playing their parents, use identical words to those they use, making it difficult for them to claim subsequently that their children *'never listen to me'*.

Cross-fostering

This technique promotes new experiences and related perspective changes. A child is placed ('fostered') with another family for 1 hour or longer. In return, the 'foster' family's own child is temporarily placed with the parent(s) of the first family. A task or exercise is given to each family, and in a subsequent reflection the families discuss their experiences and attempt to answer questions such as why it is more difficult to manage one's own child than the child of another family. Children can be asked to talk about what surprised them during the 'foster' time, how they reacted to certain attitudes of their 'foster' parents that they find difficult to tolerate from their own parents and what they missed that their parents usually do and why. When managing the children of other families, many parents discover hidden or long-forgotten competencies which they can use later with their own children.

Video feedback

Recording interactions audio-visually can be used to great effect, as one sees oneself, one's family and others from a different perspective. This can help to pinpoint strengths and difficulties, and, in conversations with other families in a reflective setting, new ideas for change can emerge. It can also be particularly helpful to view and discuss recordings of problematic situations in a group setting. Video recordings can not only be made during MFT sessions, but families can also be encouraged to film situations and interactions they regard as important at home on their mobile phones and bring them to a MFT session for general viewing. Mentalizing techniques are particularly useful for video feedback meetings (see Chapter 4). It starts with observing a sequence and recounting what one is imagining may be happening in a particular interaction. The sequence can be freeze-framed, and everyone can speculate about what might be going on in any of the protagonists during that scene and, following this, what feelings this may invoke in them themselves.

Collaborative psychoeducation

Traditional psychoeducation, consisting of lecturing a group of people or families about a particular subject, like a disorder or illness and its treatment, does not fit well with the systemic paradigm, as it relies on an expert who 'knows it all' and on an audience which is viewed as knowing rather little or nothing. In a multi-family group of 25–30 people there is likely to be plenty of experience and expertise, and if one creates a context where this can be pooled, then this can open the door to families becoming partners in promoting any form of new learning. This can be done by forming small buzz groups, with each formulating their ideas and, once they have done so, presenting these in turn to the large group. If there are any gaps in specific facts or data, group members can access the Internet and see whether these can be filled with information available there. One of the practitioners' roles is to encourage the critical evaluation of information obtained via Internet sources and how to judge what is trustworthy information and what not. Once each group has had their say, consideration can be given to getting one or two group members to bring all this together and deliver a formal lecture. The following example illustrates how collaborative psychoeducation can be introduced.

'*Dear families, all of you here in this room have very similar disorders/illnesses/ difficulties. If one does have such illnesses, one needs to know the facts, for example, the symptoms, the reason for treatments, the medication and its side effects and how the body responds, not to mention what those near and dear can do to help or signs that a relapse might be eminent. Since these are illnesses, some of you may well think that only doctors know all about it, but that isn't true in our experience. We have found that if you families put all your heads together and pool what you know, then your expertise can help us to understand what it is like to live with the illness. Who here knows something about anorexia nervosa – what is it? What do you know about its causes and treatment? Just say or shout out aloud what you know, and I will write this up on a flip chart. . . '.* Later: '*Well, there are plenty of ideas here . . . which of you would like to give a formal lecture on this subject? Here is a white coat – we need a professor (encourage children/teenagers) to sum it all up – so much easier to do so in the white coat of the expert.*' Later: '*Which of your questions have still not been answered? Who might have the relevant information? How could you get it? Here is a laptop and the Internet, just in case you might want to use it*'.

Chapter 4

Mentalizing and MFT

A match made in heaven?

What is mentalizing?

Mentalizing is an imaginative activity that seeks to interpret human behaviours in terms of intentional mental states. It is an innate capacity that develops most easily in the context of relatively secure and consistent caregiving relationships and at different rates and in different ways, depending on each individual's culture, social situation and life events. Some disorders may impact the development of mentalizing, but that does not mean that people with such disorders are unable to mentalize. Imagination underpins mentalizing and enables us to intuit the thoughts, feelings and intentions of those around us and thereby make sense of their actions, just as we at the same time organize our own subjective experiences. Mentalizing is about paying attention to and reflecting on your own mental state and the mental state of other people. It is important for representing, communicating and regulating feelings and belief states linked to our wishes and desires and whether they are being met, threatened or frustrated.

We mentalize when we try to perceive the internal psychological state in ourselves and in other people and their interactions differently and appropriately. Often we do this automatically and 'preconsciously', and we call this *implicit* mentalizing. At other times we will do so deliberately or *explicitly*, when we consciously try to put into words mental states – feelings, intentions, needs, attitudes, evaluations, motives, fantasies and thoughts. Effective mentalizing is a bit of 'hit and miss', as sometimes we succeed better and sometimes less so. This is not all that surprising, as emotional states can only be roughly grasped – not only in others but also in oneself. Furthermore, mentalizing is a fragile capacity. When we are very emotionally aroused, our frontal lobe – which is where an important part of our mentalizing takes place – shuts down like a computer, and people can 'no longer see the forest for the trees' or are plainly 'seeing red'. To then ask highly aroused group members to mentalize themselves and others is unlikely to be productive.

There are also considerable individual differences and fluctuations in how capable of effective mentalizing people are, how easy they find it, how quickly they can regain mentalizing when it has been temporarily lost and how rigid and inflexible mentalizing can become. Misinterpretations can lead to misunderstandings, and

DOI: 10.4324/9781003442424-4

these in turn to impulsive and confused interactions in which we do not see the others as they are, and neither do they see us. However, such breaks in mentalizing happen to a greater or lesser degree in all relationships and, when returned to and repaired, misunderstandings can strengthen mentalizing capacity and relationships.

The terms 'mentalization' and 'mentalizing' were first introduced into the psychotherapeutic world by French psychoanalysts some three decades ago (Marty, 1991), albeit with different meanings than those developed by Peter Fonagy and colleagues in London (Fonagy et al., 1991). The goal of pure 'mentalization-based' or 'mentalization-supportive' or 'mentalization-promoting' therapy – all three terms are currently used interchangeably – is simply to stimulate and optimize 'mentalization'. However, this somewhat unfortunate word ('mentalization') sounds as if one is talking about a result or even a product. The verb 'to mentalize', on the other hand, is probably more appropriate since it refers to an active inter-subjective process, containing both a self-reflective and an interpersonal component and thus making it relevant for all kinds of work with groups, including MFT, social networks and organizations (Asen et al., 2019).

Mentalization theory and practice is a multi-pillared bridging concept that intersects and connects with other approaches to psychotherapy, whether client-centred, cognitive, dialectical-behavioural, mindfulness-based or systemic. It is possible to view the mentalization-inspired or -oriented stance and the resulting interventions as an important addition to already existing family systemic approaches (Asen & Fonagy, 2021). Family work, that is, the direct 'live' work with important attachment figures, be that in a single- or multi-family context, is a natural context for the promotion of mentalizing. The multi-family setting offers unique opportunities to practice mentalizing with and on other families.

Mentalization-based theories and practices have inspired many systemic practitioners over the past decade and somehow bridged the gap that used to exist between the psychodynamic and systemic worlds and their therapies (Asen & Fonagy, 2012a). Mentalization-inspired systemic therapy (MIST) aims to enhance mentalizing in order to open a person to improved social communication and interaction not only within the family but also in other social settings, and it thereby aims to increase openness to learning and epistemic trust (Fonagy et al., 2015). Epistemic trust can be defined as the confidence and trust in the information about the social world that we receive from another person, be that a teacher, a parent or another significant person. When we can take in what others communicate to us as having personal relevance, our ability to adapt in the face of challenging situations is enhanced. The therapeutic focus of MIST is on encouraging the natural process for solving social problems by genuinely considering each other's experiences and points of view. It is the experience of feeling one's perspective of reality is aligned with another's which improves one's confidence in the value of engaging with perspective taking as a whole. In a family context, such an experience can open the mind of each family member to the possibility of learning and discovering something relevant to them within the family.

In a multi-family group, the potential therapeutic benefit of such experience is amplified, as there will be a majority of families who feel, on some level, connected with one another. The concept of the 'we-mode' (Tuomela, 2006; Gallotti & Frith, 2013) is relevant here: it asserts that the mere presence of others (i.e., the social context) improves a person's potential for mentalizing by broadening their aware- ness of the options for action and for generating new solutions. Co-representing the viewpoints of others and generating a 'psychological collective' by joining forces leads to the emerging sense of 'we-ness', of shared perspectives and shared minds, which is at the heart of relational mentalizing and which powers MFT. Families and their members can see themselves and their interactions and communications mirrored in other families. This is much more likely to happen when families have similar issues, and this is also one of the main reasons for bringing families with 'related' disorders together. Thus, in this benign social environment, there are increased opportunities for group members to experience feeling seen and under- stood and to be exposed to a broader range of perspectives, building epistemic trust and openness to social learning. Furthermore, MFT provides families with an opportunity to practice and experience effective mentalizing, as it invites them to pay attention to other families and to explicitly speculate about their mental states. As families get to know each other and once sufficient group cohesion is estab- lished, they are increasingly able to hear their own mental states commented on by other group members, and this enables them to reflect on how they are experienced by other families and their members.

Mentalization-informed practitioners do not aim primarily to help families to find pragmatic solutions to problems but rather to stimulate and promote effective mentalizing and to assist families and their members to recover their mentalizing capacity when this is blocked. Such blocks can, for example, include suddenly and unexpectedly refusing to answer a question, going 'blank' or inadvertently or deliberately misunderstanding what another family member has said. The removal of blocks can help a family and its members to find its very own solution or a way forward and, over time, lead them to develop a better understanding of themselves and each other.

Mentalizing dimensions

Four dimensions of mentalizing can be described, which are polar opposites (Fonagy & Luyten, 2009). One of these dimensions has already been referred to, 'implicit' and 'explicit' (automatic and controlled) mentalizing. Most mentalizing takes place on an implicit level until there is a need to share or to better understand internal states. Another dimension is the focus on 'internal' as opposed to 'exter- nal' processes: what is happening mentally and emotionally inside people, in their heads and bellies, so to speak, and what is apparent on the outside. Focusing pri- marily on reading facial expressions and body language can run the risk of neglect- ing internal mental states and vice versa. The third dimension is the difference between 'self-oriented' and 'other-oriented' mentalizing. Some people find it easier to mentalize the emotional states of others and less easy to reflect on their own experience. Others can be predominantly self-focused. The fourth dimension of mentalizing consists of the poles 'cognitive' and 'affective': at one pole of this spectrum, we have the exclusive focus on rational understanding and logic, and at the other end of the spectrum is the over-preoccupation with affect.

It is optimal when people can move flexibly between these poles: then they can usually automatically and quickly implicitly mentalize when everything is going well and switch to explicit mentalizing when more attention is required. Flexible mentalizers are able to focus temporarily on internal processes (needs, desires, beliefs) but also focus on external aspects (actions, facial expressions, body language); they can illuminate their own feelings in a self-oriented manner and at other times in an other-oriented manner. Flexible mentalizers have both a good cognitive and emotional understanding of mental processes and bring these understandings together. However, if people are predominantly fixed on one pole of one or more of the mentalizing dimensions, their ability to mentalize is limited. Therapeutic interventions try to help individuals and families move flexibly between both poles of these four dimensions and also to address the 'land in between'. It's a matter of balancing.

Balancing mentalizing dimensions in MFT

The structural frame of MFT and its emphasis on context making and context changing means that the approach provides continual opportunities to balance dimensions of mentalizing. Practitioners themselves are walking a tightrope, continuously adjusting and re-adjusting the balance via different interventions in order to promote mentalizing in the group. It can look like this:

- When it's too cognitive in the group, the practitioners can raise arousal by bringing an emotional focus into the conversation or by introducing an activity that will raise affect and/or energy. Conversely, when arousal is too high, an activity that demands cognitive attention or focuses on self-regulation can be introduced;
- Implicit mentalizing can be made explicit when appropriate, either via discussions about how different activities were experienced and what can be transferred home, by connecting groups and sub-groups to make sense of interactions or behaviours within the group or by the use of specific techniques – like the following mentalization-supporting questions;
- If the focus is too external, practitioners can stimulate interest in internal mental processes, for example, by introducing an activity that shifts group member's attention onto their bodies. Conversely, an activity that demands close attention to other people, or the wider context, can shift the focus outwards;
- When group members are overly fixated on others, self-focused interventions may be used, such as pausing a current activity or discussion and engaging

people in short, individual tasks. Conversely, a group-connecting activity can be used to shift the focus from self to other.

Focusing excessively on explicit mentalizing, as can be the way with some thera-peutic approaches, can become a rigid formula and invite 'pseudo-mentalizing', also known as 'rambling'. However, context shifting to promote mentalizing in the ways described previously requires that families help each other to regain and develop their mentalizing capacity in 'real time', and the practitioners can observe this process and only need to intervene when non-mentalizing takes over.

As there is considerable variety in people's capacity to mentalize generally, and as 'triggers' to non-mentalizing can also vary, it is unlikely that, at any given time, the whole group will be 'positioned' at one end of any of the given mentalizing dimensions. However, it is often the case that a significant number of group mem-bers will become 'unbalanced' in similar directions and can then be 'rebalanced' in the ways described previously. In these instances, those group members who have managed to maintain their mentalizing capacity can be used to help those who have not. Where unbalanced mentalizing is identified on a more individual or single-family level, the practitioners' intervention should reflect this by intervening at an individual or sub-group rather than whole-group level. If practitioners have managed to create a context where a group, sub-group or individual does regain their mentalizing capacity, it is important to go on and think with the group, family or individual what they might have learnt from the process and how they might transfer this learning outside the group.

MFT as an emotional regulator

While a certain level of arousal is therapeutically important to stimulate new pro-cesses, too much arousal temporarily impairs the ability to mentalize. In addition to the balancing interventions described previously and the specific mentalizing techniques described subsequently, there are several components of MFT that can be particularly effective with regard to creating a helpful emotional 'distance' from loaded issues. Such distance allows families to engage with potentially highly emotive topics in a more regulated way, making effective mentalizing more likely. One of the reasons why audiovisual recording of multi-family group work can be so helpful is precisely this: a few hours or days later, one can see oneself and others on the screen with more peace of mind and mentalize oneself and others to change one's behaviour and perspectives or at least be open to it. Audio-visual recording of family and group interactions enable retrospection through later video feedback in the group context, when one's own excitement has subsided and effective men-talization can begin again. Reflective teams (see Chapter 3) can work in a similar way in that feedback is provided while the family member is in a more regulated position.

MFT also enables families to observe attachment behaviours in other fami-lies from a 'safe' distance and to register differences and similarities to their own behaviours. This is a more benign and less fearful experience than immediately focusing on one's own family bonding and attachment issues, as this tends to evoke high levels of arousal, which can block effective mentalizing. Inter-family cross-fostering procedures allow children and parents to sit in on a 'strange' family and then mentalize their experiences and bonding experiences in their own family. Bonding and attachment issues can then also be discussed in a group context, and comparisons with other families open up new perspectives.

The playful nature of MFT activities and exercises can in themselves create a safe emotional distance and are an ideal context for working on potentially highly emotive and/or usually avoided topics together with parents and children. In addition to the relative ease of doing something together in the playful activities, their 'as if' mode enables parents and children to have new perspectives and experiences. With the variety of activities, there is a high probability that typical problematic family interactions and relationships will present or develop spontaneously. This creates an opportunity for a natural and more attuned response than if the practitioners were asking families to talk about or show them some of their difficulties, as is often the case in traditional single-family therapy. Such conversations can often lead to children getting bored and losing interest.

Finally, the fact that the practitioners aim to de-centralize themselves and to create contexts where families help one another can be emotionally regulating. For example, rather than simply responding to the perceived needs of the group, the practitioners can recruit some group members to help them 'take the temperature' and make decisions about what is needed. This can be done in a playful way by, for example, asking parents to place a stethoscope on their child's head and abdomen to 'listen' to what is 'on their mind' and their 'gut feelings'.

Aims and techniques of mentalization-informed-systemic therapy

The main focus of mentalization-informed-systemic therapy is on the behaviour and relationship patterns existing between family members (Asen & Fonagy, 2021). These can only be changed in the long term if the thoughts and feelings of the individual and the relationships between family members are addressed in a differentiated manner. Thus, MIST practitioners acknowledge different points of view, give them positive connotations and repeatedly and explicitly check that they have correctly understood what each individual means, thinks and feels. The practitioners show that they can't really know how a family or group member is feeling without asking a question designed to find out. Mentalization-focused interventions move from asking questions of orientation to creating a consensual, understandable use of language that makes it possible to talk about mental states, especially affects (Asen & Fonagy, 2012a). When something is unclear, mentalization-oriented therapists ask for clarification and reflection, using the sequence: 'interrupt – repeat – explore – reflect'. This means pausing discussions to reflect, to examine what is happening – or has happened – in the 'here and now', to explore feelings and opinions and then to reflect on them. When non-mentalizing processes take over, one can 'rewind' and check at which point effective mentalizing was deteriorating or when it was lost. MIST practitioners think that by encouraging and removing obstacles to family members' ability to think about each individual's mental state (including their own), many family problems can be reduced or resolved.

However, it is important to state that more effective mentalizing is a way to understand relationship difficulties and to be able to deal with them better, as well as to regulate affects more effectively. There is no 'perfect' mentalizing, since perfection simply does not fit into the mentalizing concept, and what MIST practitioners aim for is to identify, highlight, promote and support mentalizing that is 'good enough'. It is a collaborative search for new understanding, for different perspectives, for mutual respect, compassion, consideration and, above all, for feeling understood. In other words, effective mentalizing is not a simple, quickly achievable state but a long, perhaps never-ending, journey with new goals being set again and again. Mentalizing can always only be an attempt to better understand one's own world and the world of others, as errors and misunderstandings are part of interpersonal encounters from which we can learn a lot about ourselves and others.

Mentalization-informed systemic practitioners generally see themselves in their work as being 'benevolently curious' (Cecchin, 1987), with a genuine and empathetic interest in other people and their histories. They are aware of their prejudices and try not to let them flow into their therapeutic work but are open to feedback and take responsibility for repairing things when they inevitably do. MIST practitioners aim to be humble about their own expertise and adopt a 'not-knowing' position, also known as the 'Socratic stance', which also permits expressing doubts about the degree of 'truth' or validity of their own perceptions, perspectives and opinions. The Greek philosopher Socrates focused on asking his students a series of open-ended questions to promote reflection and awakening knowledge which had been previously outside of their awareness. This method enabled them to open up new perspectives and reach their own conclusions rather than being told what these should be by the questioner. Similarly, MIST practitioners take the time to question, identify, name, accept and explicitly legitimize the different perspectives of each family member, young and old. They demonstrate that they can change their own perspectives through better understanding. MIST practitioners avoid having to understand what seems incomprehensible and try to find and gain understanding through reflective questions, focusing on detailed descriptions mental states and avoiding 'why' questions. They do not interpret or construe what might be 'behind' family members' communications, even when it is more than tempting. MIST practitioners explicitly focus on the changing and potentially changeable mental states. They intervene specifically when encountering mentalization difficulties and systematically block non-mentalizing interactions and communications. They are constantly on the lookout for effective mentalizing, working hard to promote and generalize mentalizing beyond their observation. This 'way of being', sometimes referred to as 'the mentalizing stance', is concordant with a

MFT approach and should be adopted by practitioners. In fact, the MFT setting often allows implementation of the mentalizing stance beyond that which can be achieved when undertaking single-family work. This is because it explicitly places a high value on the family's sense of agency in terms of their resources and capacity to support one another rather than being dependent on the input by an 'expert'. Having agency ascribed and strengths valued in an experiential 'real time' way promotes epistemic trust and is an extension of the mentalizing stance that is hard to achieve so effectively in single-family work. Having their minds being 'online' all the time is not an easy task for practitioners, as their own feelings, prejudices and other states of mind can divert focus and attention. Thus, it is to be expected that a practitioner's mentalizing capacity will be compromised numerous times throughout a busy, dynamic MFT group. Just like the families, the aim is for the practitioners to maintain 'good enough' mentalizing and to recognize when this has gone 'offline'. This is one reason multi-family groups are always run by two practitioners who can support and regulate one another.

The mentalizing spiral

In MFT, as indeed in single-family work, practitioners can choose to become attentive to any emerging opportunities for fostering a mentalizing atmosphere and encourage group members to speculate about the mental states of others, followed by discussions of these speculations. This process aims to initiate a dynamic of 'mind-storming', characterized by ongoing checking of whether other group members perceive mental states in similar or different ways. The concept of the mentalizing spiral (Figure 4.1) serves as a fitting metaphor for this approach. However, unlike a downward spiral, which is marked by a self-perpetuating cycle of negative behaviours, thoughts and feelings that lead to worsening situations, the mentalizing spiral represents a progressively ascending and expanding curve around a central mentalizing axis. Going round it a few times enables increasingly sophisticated interventions and thus reflects progression. Each new level of this spiral is a response to a stimulus from the previous level, resembling a map with multiple routes towards more effective mentalizing. It's a practical tool for discovering new ways to move beyond current stalemates. A mentalizing spiral is created when practitioners punctuate an interaction or conversation, followed by a series of questions that prompt group members to reflect in a mentalizing manner. The practitioners invite group members to focus on the present moment within, for example, a group activity or during a single-family exercise, encouraging them to conjecture about their own and others' thoughts and feelings. This invitation to mentalize, along with the subsequent responses, generates a spiralling process of 'mind-storming', accompanied by a continuous checking for congruence or divergence in the perception of mental states.

The goal of focusing on a particular interaction sequence is to engage group members in considering the mental states of everyone involved, including themselves.

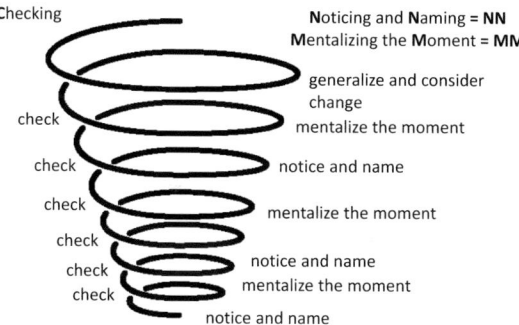

Figure 4.1 The mentalizing spiral

By mentally pausing, rewinding and revisiting a specific interaction sequence, practitioners can facilitate the development of multiple meta-perspectives, enhancing effective mentalizing. Practitioners first observe and name a communication or interaction and then immediately check this observation. This is followed by prompting group members to mentalize the moment, encouraging them to imagine the mental states and relationships of those involved in a specific interaction. The emphasis is placed on attributing mental states, with the practitioners highlighting particular descriptions, checking and verifying their own understanding and then urging group members to mentalize these new moments.

This recursive process of progressing along the upward spiral is the core therapeutic activity, rather than aiming to reach a definitive 'truth' about the potential underlying causes for the described interaction. By methodically moving from one mentalizing moment to the next and checking the perceptions of all involved, practitioners can prevent 'mindless' escalations. Highlighting problematic interaction sequences effectively pauses potential escalations, and the process of mentally rewinding and reviewing these sequences generates a series of meta-perspectives, further fostering effective mentalizing. This approach not only aids in understanding each other's perspectives but also helps in maintaining control over the therapy process, avoiding the common experience of situations spiralling out of control.

As in the 'five-step model' (see previously), the first phase of the mentalizing spiral (Figure 4.2) focuses on the cautious 'noting and naming' of observed intra- or inter-family interactions. The following are a few examples of how this can be done:

'I just noticed that you are both arguing very loudly and that Emily and Bill are turning their faces to the wall';
'I have the feeling that the women in this group want to think about shame and that the men here try anything to avoid getting involved in this discussion'

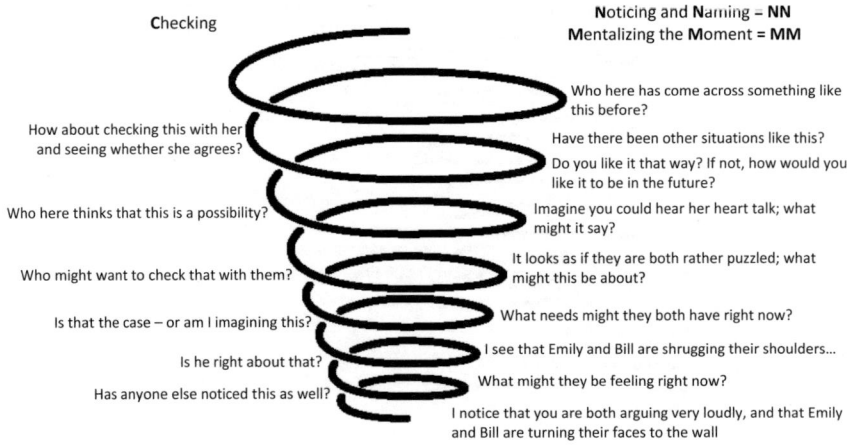

Figure 4.2 The mentalizing spiral in action

'I am not sure I am right, but I get the impression seems that some people here believe that conflicts in the family should never be discussed in front of everyone'.

Checking out and securing consensus, *'Has anyone else noticed this as well?'*, about this description is again rather similar to the second step of the five-step model. In a multi-family group, the checking is also an invitation to everyone to contribute their own observations, though, with many participants, finding consensus can be even more difficult than in a single-family session. But in the end, it is helpful because the goal of mentalization-informed work is not to create a consensus but to stimulate curiosity and to be able to read and understand mental states in oneself and others better via mentalizing conversations. If participants state that they have no idea what the practitioners are talking about, then such feedback should prompt them to consider the usefulness or accuracy of their observations or consider that noting and naming may be too challenging for some at this point. Practitioners may then say: *'We seem to be quite wrong, or maybe we have lost the plot? Help us: what might have happened to us that we experienced it so differently? Who can help us?'*

The purpose of highlighting a particular interaction sequence is to engage the group members to engage in joint attention (a necessary prerequisite for mentalization) and focus on everyone's minds, including their own. By mentally rewinding and reviewing a specific sequence in this way, a series of meta-perspectives can be generated, which can further promote effective mentalizing. Specific examples of mentalization-stimulating interventions are described subsequently, in concrete and direct language.

'What do you think it's all about? What might be going on in Anna? What feelings might prompt them to behave this way? And how does that affect others here? What do you think about when you witness something like this? Have you ever been in a situation like this?'

'We want to ask you, all the men here, what must be going on in the mothers' minds when you hear that one shouldn't talk about shame in front of everyone? If you could see thought bubbles above mothers' heads, what would they say?'

'There seems to be total radio silence from all the families here when it comes to figuring out how conflicts arise. What could be the concerns of the participants here that you don't want to or can't talk about conflicts in your family?'

'What do you think/make of what just happened here?'

'What do you think about this? And what did you think and feel about this situation?'

'Why do you think the kids' reaction was totally different than the parents'?'

'What might the father have been thinking when he suddenly became angry/dismissive/anxious? What could his motives be?

'What do you think the child (the mother/father) would have expected from you (the parents) – or maybe even needed?'

'What do you think Mr. Mayer was thinking; what was going on in his wife's head (or elsewhere)? Who can help him there?'

'And if that were the case, what feelings or needs would that have triggered in Ms. Mayer?'

'How can children deal with apparently non-understandable behaviour from their parents?'

'How can children judge what is, and is not, acceptable and 'normal' parenting behaviour?'

'How do such assessments develop?'

'And whose responsibility is it to talk to the child and understand their perspective?'

At some point, the practitioners may ask to link the 'here-and-now' mental states to other situations that may have arisen in the course of ordinary family life situations. This marks the second phase of the mentalizing spiral. Practitioners can help group members to generalize by moving away from a specific interaction that had stimulated mentalizing to more general observations and thoughts about how similar patterns of interaction often develop in the home and how to understand the feelings triggered, by stating: *'We've experienced a bit here how difficult it can be to talk about conflicts. Who knows that from home?'* Linking the specifics of acute interaction to more general interaction patterns unfolding at home or in other 'real-life' contexts is key to stabilizing mentalizing within the system, be that a family, a multi-family group or indeed an institution. Asking generalizing questions (see examples subsequently) may achieve this: *'Have you noticed whether things like this are also sometimes happening at home or elsewhere?'* This phase represents the broadening of the upper parts of the mentalizing spiral, as the perspectives of group members expand. The focus shifts from the specific interaction that initially stimulated mentalizing to broader observations and reflections on how similar interaction patterns commonly emerge at home or elsewhere and understanding the emotions these interactions evoke. Linking the specifics of live, immediate interactions to more general patterns that unfold in other 'real-life' contexts is crucial for maintaining stable mentalizing both in the group and beyond. The aim of this phase of the mentalizing spiral is to generate new thoughts connected to potential actions. The objective is to use mentalizing as a pathway to solutions, not to convince group members or an entire family to embrace a particular solution. This approach helps in not only understanding the dynamics of the interactions but also in exploring alternative ways of responding to similar situations in the future. By recognizing these patterns and their associated feelings, group members can develop more effective ways of interacting and responding to each other. Thus, the practitioner can notice and name the following: '*I can see that Emily and Bill think that they should be allowed to come clean about not wanting to join this discussion and that the rest of the group should accept this. I think it is possible that they both feel under a lot of pressure. Have I got that right? And what might be in the minds of other group members? Why don't you all talk about that now . . . ?*'

Five steps and/or mentalizing spiral?

The five-step model (see Chapter 3) is primarily a goal- and change-focused approach. It can be adapted if one wants to use a primarily mentalization-informed approach – which is not after achieving specific goals and related changes but insists that it is the continuous and recursive process of mentalizing, going round and round, in a spiralling motion as it were, that is therapeutic in its own right. The practitioners consciously slow down the pace of multi-family work and focus on mental states but do not, as in the five-step model, invite families to immediately move on to the 'wish for change'. Mentalizing the moment, such as a mother's visible state of excitement or the paralysis of a group of father to talk about intra-family conflicts, means focusing on what may be experienced in the here and now. The practitioners' task is to keep the focus on mental states rather than on quick-seeming 'solutions'. Often, therefore, they have to 'note and name' again or maybe even in a different way and repeatedly seek whether there is a consensus. It is this repetitive rewinding and fast-forwarding which constitutes the mentalizing spiral. Example: '*I notice that everyone in the Smith family shook their heads when I said that the families here simply cannot or do not want to talk about their conflicts. Did others here notice this too? What might be going on in the different heads of the Smith family right now? Who wants to speculate here? And now I realize that everyone is paralyzed . . . maybe I said something that is totally off the mark? Can someone help me here? What do you think is on my mind? What feelings and needs might I have right now?*'

In MFT one can use both the mentalizing spiral and the five-step model. In the case of the latter, one of the goals is to focus on making concrete changes and to consider taking specific steps to achieve these. The five-step model is an action-oriented intervention tool, whereas the mentalizing spiral is a reflexive one. Steps suggest a linear progression and are often an important prerequisite for promoting sustainable actions. Spirals, on the other hand, are recursive and circular in nature and thus promote reflective processes.

From structure to content to process

MFT provides an excellent setting for the promotion and recovery of mentalizing. However, it is only likely to be effective as such if the practitioners themselves are able to maintain and recover their own mentalizing capacities throughout the group work, making well-attuned and balanced contexts for families. This can be a challenge due to the broad range of needs and abilities of families and the dynamic nature of multi-family groups, which can sometimes feel like (organized!) chaos. Practitioners often make it explicit when their own capacity to mentalize has temporarily gone offline and when they need to pause or use their co-therapist or go back to understand something better, and this is something that also tends to work well in multi-family groups, with the practitioners recruiting the support of the families to get them back on track. A particular challenge is making contexts that are accessible to, and engaging for, both children and adults. Activities involving the contribution of children should always be developmentally accessible to the youngest child involved in the activity. Higher-level mentalizing interventions, such as some of the mentalizing questions and the use of the mentalizing spiral, can be inaccessible to children and also to some parents and carers. It is the role of the practitioners to continually monitor the accessibility of the interventions they are offering and, if need be, change the context in order to ensure that *all* group members feel 'seen' and heard.

Chapter 5

Making contexts for interventions

Setting up MFT projects

Deciding to set up an MFT project is one thing; implementing it is another matter. The idea may be attractive, but the reality of converting it into practice is usually not without obstacles. When people attend MFT workshops or training courses, they are often eager to start a new project, and they may have already a target group of families in mind. For example, practitioners working in child and adolescent mental health services may get excited by the idea of providing MFT for families with a child diagnosed with ADHD, ASD, Tourette's syndrome or conduct disorder. If they work mostly with adolescents, they may consider a project with suicidal or eating-disordered teenagers and their families. Practitioners working in schools may think about starting MFT for families where a child is not attending school or for disruptive pupils. Practitioners working in social care may want to focus on families presenting with suspected or confirmed child abuse and neglect. Obviously, institutional dynamics and political health priorities will also play a role as to which particular disorder or problems to focus on. There are also practitioners who want to practice MFT but who do not have a clear focus of work in mind.

Practitioners first experimenting with MFT are well advised to start using the approach with what appear to be 'easier' families and not with families who have been struggling for years with chronic problems or disorders that have not responded to a wide range of previous treatment attempts. Unfortunately, it is a not at all uncommon that whenever one promotes a new approach and invites referrals, one tends to receive the most seemingly 'impossible' cases, particularly from sceptical colleagues. MFT is unlikely to work when everything else has failed. We recommend that clinicians start with small and discrete MFT projects, initially funded from existing resources, rather than making a plea for up-front pump-prime funding, which usually is not forthcoming. Using the financial argument as an excuse for being unable to start MFT is not uncommon but hardly credible, particularly if one considers that two staff can treat up to eight families at the same time. A pilot project can encourage staff to acquire confidence and competencies, and it can also serve to convince colleagues and managers at a later stage to invest in MFT. At the outset it is best *not* to replace an already existing project with a new MFT venture, as

DOI: 10.4324/9781003442424-5

institutional resistance may give it a bad start. MFT should rather be thought of as an 'add-on', being implemented to assist already good work rather than putting itself at risk by being perceived as a potential competitor. Another consideration as to what type of families to work with is the age of the 'identified' problem carrier. It is generally easier to start MFT with families containing younger children. Teenagers are much more difficult to motivate to attend therapy groups together with their parents.

Convincing management and colleagues

Most MFT projects take place in institutional settings, be that in education, health or social care. Here both the fear of, and enthusiasm for, implementing an exciting new project tend to be bedfellows, and mentalizing managers and colleagues as well as oneself and one's potential team members is almost essential to avoid disappointments and eventual failure. When first vetting the idea of starting a bespoke MFT project with managers, one needs to be mindful of how to 'sell' it. Managers tend to think of financial, reputational and risk issues and often want a business plan. They are also likely to ask for the evidence base of a new approach. Other practitioners and colleagues from the same service or institution may feel excluded or even threatened and can be worried about the implications of a new project for their own work, fearing that their own work or service could be adversely affected if the project were to be successful. And, if the new MFT project turns out to be successful, they may be afraid that a new model of work might clash with their own training and therapeutic doctrine. Dealing with predictable resistances and fears is part of the preparation for MFT work. Helpful arguments for using MFT include, for example, that it is not financially expensive and cheaper than other approaches. There is also a 'good enough' evidence base that MFT works for different presentations and disorders, that it has very low attrition rates (see Chapter 2) and that its negative side effects are negligible. Another argument that may be useful is that MFT lends itself very much to dealing with long waiting lists (see Chapter 8).

For practitioners embarking on MFT it may be prudent to give a presentation to management and colleagues prior to starting the actual work, outlining its theory, practice and evidence base. It is important to adopt a position of humility when doing so and not to exaggerate the efficacy of MFT. It may also be wise to report at regular intervals on the work in progress and not to hide any problems or shortcomings of the approach. If there are problems with recruitment or treatment dropouts, one can explain to managers and colleagues why these might have happened and ask for their perspectives and ideas. Total transparency about the scope and limitations of the work, including negative outcomes, pays off, as does asking explicitly for advice and help from colleagues and managers.

Recruiting families

The recruitment of families to a new MFT project can only begin once the practitioners are clear what the target group of families and the main work focus are and once there is institutional support for the project. Assuming the latter has been obtained, a decision needs to be made about what to call the MFT project, as this helps families and their members make up their minds about joining. The more memorable and non-stigmatizing the group name or title is, the better. Examples are: Early Days (for young parents with babies), Kidstime (for young carers and their psychiatrically ill parents), No Kids in the Middle (for high-conflict families), Family School (for excluded pupils and their carers) or Gut Feelings (for families with obesity issues). However, it can be quite a task to find appropriate names or titles for projects: the term Family Day Unit, for example, was coined for a bespoke project for 'multi-problem families' which is not how the families would have described themselves, hence the selection of a neutral term. However, this is not to say that some of the very same families would not have attended an MFT project called Tackling Family Violence (which has been a successful MFT project!), yet others, being in denial, would simply not do so. MFT projects for Multi-Stressed Families (Overbeek et al., 2021; van Beek et al., 2023) is a much more catchy title for the very same families, and successful work continues to be done with them (see Chapter 9).

MFT works best if there is a minimum of four families, as with fewer families, there is a risk that due to illness or other reasons for occasional non-attendance, there will at times be only two or sometimes only one family present, not a good number for multi-family group work! One way of recruiting families for MFT is to advertise the new project among colleagues and related institutions. Another recruitment path is to encourage families already known to the practitioners and/ or service. Some practitioners may find it difficult to accommodate families and/ or their individual members with whom they have already an ongoing therapeutic relationship. This should not be an obstacle to include them in MFT if the practitioners explain the boundaries and that they work in the group for *everyone* and have to be even handed as to whom they pay their attention to. In the single-family meetings that precede the first MFT session, this issue can be addressed. In the scenario of practitioners having only been able to identify two suitable families for a specific MFT project, they could consider convening at least a one-off 'two-family meeting' by asking each family whether they would like to meet another family who has similar issues. This could be the beginning of generating enough interest in other families over time if one is on the lookout for similar pairings of families, leading eventually to the recruitment of a sufficient number of families to form a functioning MFT group.

Staffing issues and work settings

Generally, most MFT work can be carried out by two practitioners, though having potentially three practitioners available for the work allows for coverage during sickness leave or holidays. Having too many staff present, including trainees, can have a paralyzing effect on families, who may feel outnumbered by professionals. It may also pose a problem for practitioners and other staff members to find a useful role and not succumb to the temptation 'to do something' merely to justify one's very presence. Apart from staff, MFT also requires the use of a room big enough to accommodate six to eight families. One room only may be sufficient for carrying out MFT projects which take place for two to three hours on a fortnightly or monthly basis. MFT work in day clinic settings requires a minimum of two large rooms.

MFT which takes place for two to three hours at fortnightly or less frequent intervals is generally acceptable for most working parents. For families requiring whole-day attendances over months, there are often problems with adults taking that much time off work. Some take annual leave, others work shifts or, in a two-parent family, take it in turn to attend. If MFT sessions are scheduled in the late afternoons, early evenings or even on weekends, 'significant others', including working parents, extended family and supporters, can attend at least some of the MFT sessions. It is also important to point out that not every family member needs to attend each MFT session, as this may not be realistic and lead to a false picture. The time-honoured concept that the 'whole family' needs to attend family therapy does not reflect the reality of the lives of many families. For example, teenagers who are the sibling(s) of a 'problem child' will often not want to commit themselves to attend all MFT sessions. They can be encouraged to be as present during MFT as they are present in the family during its waking hours. For some teenagers this would not amount to more than 10% of the time and, translated to the frequency of their MFT attendance, would mean one in ten sessions. A similar approach can be used for including semi-absent parents: they can be 'part-time MFT attenders', reflecting their seeming 'part-time status' in the family.

Language barriers and bridges

As already observed in Chapter 3, there are only very few exclusion criteria for participating in MFT, and not speaking the 'dominant' language is definitely not one of these! Using interpreters can be both helpful and problematic. It is certainly helpful for them to be present at the beginning of meetings when planning the day and also at the end of meetings when general reflections are invited and transfer tasks are discussed. This form of time- and activity-limited use of interpreters suits MFT work best. Whilst interpreters are needed for specific times and asks so that families can communicate with each other and with the practitioners, they can also get in the way and literally act as barriers between families. This is particularly the case if they are present for the whole duration of MFT groups and if they stay closely attached to their allocated family, often talking to them about other matters and thereby inadvertently impeding any naturally evolving interactions between that family and other families. Generally, it is helpful if interpreters are present for specific discussions, for example, for a planning or a reflective meeting. If so, they should sit or stand behind 'their' family so that family members can have eye contact with other group members. When, for example, two or three families do not speak English and, to make it more complicated, each speaks a different minority language, then four parallel languages will be spoken in the same room. This will make it almost impossible for everybody to be listened to and respected in what amounts to linguistic chaos. Such a scenario requires a lot of patience and tolerance on everyone's part, as each sentence uttered by group members will need to be translated backwards and forwards into each of the languages and then relayed to the group in the dominant language. For this to work to be successful, high levels of respect and self-discipline are required, as everyone must wait until the interpreters have finished their translation. Most families find this very laborious at the outset, as it slows down the group process, and it is not at all uncommon for the speakers of the dominant language to challenge *'foreign'* families openly and ask why they have not learned to speak the dominant language. It is over time that the perceived 'otherness' can become intriguing and that the group members speaking the dominant language may want to tune into the different sounds and diverse cultures from which they originate. The Tower of Babble activity can be used to thematize the issue.

MFT 'tasting events'

Most MFT work takes place in closed groups, meaning that all families start and end their attendance at the same time. An initial MFT tasting event is a suitable introduction to the work, giving families a flavour of what is to come and allowing them to make informed decisions afterwards as to whether MFT is something they wish to commit themselves to. Multi-family tasting events, which can last between one and three hours, are best scheduled late in the afternoon or in the early evening so that undecided or reluctant participants are more likely to attend. It is important that the tasting event be well structured so that families do not feel too overwhelmed or confused by a meeting with some other 20 or 30 other people unknown to them. To avoid creating unnecessary anxieties, the practitioners need to take the lead and help families and their supporters to feel as much at ease as possible.

A clear structure, apart from creating what hopefully will become a 'secure base' for the therapeutic work, will also reduce the practitioners' own anxieties. The room and general ambience have to be welcoming, with light refreshments provided. During the first 10 to 15 minutes, the MFT practitioners help families to get to know each other. This could be followed by a relatively formal presentation, explaining what MFT is and why it is helpful; this is often done by setting up the chairs in rows, like in a lecture theatre. After the presentation, which should last no longer than 15–20 minutes, questions and answers are invited. After that, small discussion groups can be formed, with each consisting of between four and five people, exchanging their thoughts and ideas about what they have heard. Each subgroup then can be asked to present any issues or further questions to the large group. This can be followed by a light-hearted ice-breaker MFT activity giving a sense that participating in MFT can be fun. One possibility is to ask participants: *'We would like you to make a poster to advertise this project. Imagine if this was the best-ever, most helpful project you had ever been to; what would the poster say? What would happen in the group? What, would make you want to come? Try and really sell it. Now, have a go, and let us see how creative you all are!'* In a final round in the large group setting, concluding reflections by both families and staff can be encouraged.

During a tasting event, families get a first experience of MFT and discover that it is not just about people sitting in a big circle and talking, as they will have been exposed to a series of different contexts, starting with a first informal, unstructured time, followed by a psychoeducational input with the group members being an audience, which is then invited to ask questions. The subsequent small-group discussions allow families to make sense of what they have heard, either each family for themselves, or two or three families and their members discussing their thoughts and ideas and exchanging these with other group members. A subsequent light-hearted MFT activity involves everyone in a playful manner. The final closing round, with everyone back in the large circle, is the last context created during a tasting event, when general feedback is invited. The introduction of 'graduate family members', adults or young persons who have previously participated in MFT work, is a very powerful tool to motivate families. It gives hope, as it provides an opportunity to listen to the experiences of individuals and families who were once in their shoes.

The first MFT session

Not all MFT projects start with a tasting event, and if such a meeting has not taken place, some of its ingredients, as described previously, would need to be employed in the first MFT session. Even when such a tasting event has taken place, it is helpful to get families to re-introduce themselves and each other. The MFT activity Speed Dating may assist and can be followed by the practitioners explaining the rationale for MFT and speculating about everyone's hopes and fears. The next part of the session can focus on a specific theme which the practitioners have identified as being relevant to the specific cohort of families, and this theme can be explored via a playful activity. Towards the end of the session, a reflective space can be created, and a homework task is given to the families. As families come to the first appointment not really knowing what to expect, it is very important to make everyone feel at ease. One way of doing so is to introduce the metaphor of 'pleading the fifth amendment' (Simic et al., 2023, p. 25), a right enshrined in the US Constitution allowing individuals to refuse to answer questions that they think might incriminate them. The practitioners explain that in MFT, every group member has the right to refuse answering questions and participating in any activity by simply saying '*I plead the fifth*'. They can add that people learn in different ways, some by listening, some by talking, some by doing, and that the way people learn can change over time, with each way of learning being potentially useful and valid (Simic et al., 2023). Introducing this metaphor usually has the effect of reducing anxiety as well as emphasizing that everyone has the right and responsibility to decide when and what personal information they wish to share. In practice, families rarely 'plead the fifth', but it encourages practitioners to ask the circular and reflexive, as well as mentalization-inducing, questions described in Chapters 3 and 4 without fearing that family members are feeling coerced into giving answers or revealing sensitive information.

There are several aims that can be addressed during the first MFT session. One aim is to connect families with families, and this can be done by asking linking questions such as: '*So this is something that you have experienced . . . has anyone in the room experienced something similar? Do you want to explain to X what it is that you have experienced?*' These questions signal that group members should begin to talk to each other rather than to the practitioners. Another aim which may have already been established in the pre-meetings with each individual family is to set up shared goals, which will also help to contribute to the evidence base for MFT work when rating regularly how and whether these have been met (see Chapter 2). This process will also help to structure future sessions around trying to monitor the goals set and/or actively addressing these. Furthermore, the themes developed during MFT sessions should reflect shared goals identified by families. A broader aim one can address in first sessions is to begin to externalize the problems or illness/disorder and to explore their impact on families and their individual members. This can be achieved via various activities, as described in Chapter 6.

Ground rules

Most institutions and work settings tend to have their own specific rules and regulations, some of which are written down and explicitly stated, while others are not. These can cover several important issues, including confidentiality, equal opportunities, anti-discriminatory practice, how to manage threats of verbal or physical violence, the use of drugs and alcohol on the premises, smoking indoors, health and safety issues and so on. Practitioners generally need to adhere to these rules and regulations when they carry out their work, no matter whether they work in schools, clinics, social services offices, in-patient units or private settings. Institutions often wrap these in rather bureaucratic language and the violation of, or non-compliance with, the rules and regulations can lead to the removal of individuals and sometimes whole families from the premises and result in a total exclusion from any further therapeutic work. There can be a tension between institution-specific rules and the rules practitioners and families might wish to establish during MFT work. MFT rules work best when they are co-constructed and regularly reviewed by families and practitioners together. In the first MFT session, practitioners can ask the group members what they believe should be the ground rules for this type of work. This should not remain a one-off question and discussion but an ongoing preoccupation, with traditional or 'old' rules being questioned and different ones introduced as new situations arise and new experiences occur.

One major issue families bring up has to do with confidentiality and boundary issues. MFT, like any other form of group work or therapy, raises very specific confidentiality issues. These issues can be more pertinent when the group is from the same geographical community, as in school-based groups, and it is thus likely that people know and see each other outside the group. The building of mutual trust is essential when wanting to share sensitive personal information with other families and their individual members. Unlike practitioners, who are bound by well-established professional confidentiality codes, families are under no such legal obligations. Yet opening up to others is essential when wanting to compare experiences, and the fear of sensitive information 'getting out' can inhibit people. To address this issue, one of the rules that can be agreed at the outset is that nobody should talk about anything they do not want to talk about and that each person is responsible for what personal information they disclose in a group setting. Practitioners may raise the question whether group members feel they need to sign a contract committing them not to talk about the group and its members outside the boundaries of the group. For some MFT practitioners, this is a must; for others, the given word counts as much as a signature on a piece of paper, which may not have much legal clout. Clearly confidentiality is an issue that benefits from ongoing discussion and reflection. MFT practitioners themselves often struggle with how to manage specific confidentiality issues, given that they are told 'confidential' information in individual or single-family meetings which is not meant to be shared with the wider group. It can be difficult for practitioners to remember what is meant to be 'public' knowledge and what not. Exploring with a family or an individual member why certain pieces of information cannot or must not be disclosed to others is important and clarifies matters for the family and for the practitioners. One way of ritualizing the importance of what is discussed in the group remaining confidential is as follows: each group member is invited to take a piece of ribbon and tie it around the doorhandle on the way into the group room. It is explained that by doing so, they are committing to keep what they hear in the group private.

Another issue that is often raised has to do with 'bad language' and swearing, particularly in front of children. This may also include examples of verbal abuse and threatened physical violence. Merely suppressing bad or unacceptable language and eventually excluding those group members is one solution and can help to provide a sanitized and orderly setting. However, it also misses the chance of working with what are ordinary day-to-day experiences for many families. Having these enacted in the MFT setting allows working with them rather than merely banning them. Yet this can be a very complicated path to negotiate, as not raising and challenging unacceptable communications or behaviours may be construed by families as staff tolerating or indeed welcoming these. Physical violence should never be tolerated, but on the very rare occasions it happens, it is better to work with its impact on everybody rather than permanently excluding the perpetrators immediately. Drug or alcohol intoxication on the premises is, of course, also not on. On the occasion when a parent attends in an intoxicated state, one can ask them, and other adults, whether it is safe for them to parent their children in such a state. The metaphor of 'driving whilst over the limit' is utilized to ask everyone whether there should be a 'parenting licence' and if so whether it should be temporarily suspended or taken away altogether. It is also possible to make use of a breathalyser to test the actual alcohol levels, and if the person shows unacceptable levels (e.g., 0.1% or above), they are asked to leave the premises and return when sober.

The Family Constitution activity can be adapted by group members to into the 'MFT Constitution', with discussions on what the most important ground rules are and how and by whom these can be enforced. There are clearly quite a few potential issues that one could 'legislate' about, and if families do not raise these, practitioners may ask whether some of the following might be relevant: the use of mobile phones and computer games; cleanliness and tidiness (who clears up whose mess?); racist, sexist and other discriminatory remarks and behaviours; responsibility for own children's behaviours; attendance of family friends or acquaintances; health and safety issues; 'talking and listening' rules; time keeping; and so on. If any of these issues are not put 'on the map' by the families themselves, the practitioners can flag some of those missed: '*Do you think we need to think about what happens if . . .?*' One can also encourage discussions on any sanctions if specific rules are broken and whether sanctions the first time round should be different from those dished out on subsequent occasions. Involving the families in devising rules and sanctions permits them to experience their own sense of agency.

Building, choosing and adjusting MFT activities

MFT sessions, no matter whether these are initial or later ones, benefit from a broad structure. Some projects will have a session-by-session structure, with special themes for each session determined prior to the work starting. Other projects will be developed and co-constructed with the families as the group unfolds. Each MFT session may nevertheless follow a somewhat similar pattern: a phase of coming together and reviewing recent events and experiences, followed by the selection of a specific theme which speaks to the issues that have brought families to participate in MFT; choosing and participating in one or more activities that illustrate the theme(s) and allow new and different perspectives and actions to emerge; and a last phase of reflecting and formulating inter-session work.

When families arrive on the day, the focus can be on how they have been doing, what the issues are for them at this point and what they might want to work on. They can start by exchanging their experiences, either in the large circle or, better still, in smaller groups. The practitioners can ask for feedback from each group and then see whether a focus on a common theme that is relevant for most families is emerging. An icebreaker activity may be chosen if there is low energy in the room. If this is not necessary, then a theme-relevant MFT activity is chosen. Many themes and activities are common to diverse conditions, like emotion regulation, family cooperation, family identity, family patterns, mentalizing processes, problem-solving and resource-seeking.

Ending MFT projects

Many MFT projects (see Chapters 8, 9 and 10) have a pre-determined structure of sessions, with specific MFT activities (see Chapter 6) and times for reflection. This includes the last MFT session. Here the main ingredients are as follows: acknowledging the 'journey' to date and the many useful contributions made by each group members. This can be done in a ritualized way by issuing certificates during a little festive celebration. Various MFT activities can be used to elicit feedback from group members (e.g., Popping Balloons). Thinking about the transfer of the experiences and learning during MFT is another important aspect of the last session. This can be done in the form of the task of each family imagining coming together one year later and telling each other what they might report about their family life is and how it has been helped by participating in the group. Another way of structuring the last day of an MFT project is to give the following instruction at the beginning of the last day, demonstrating to families that it is in their power to create meaningful contexts for addressing specific issues: '*Today is our last MFT day. We want you to pretend that we, the practitioners, are not able, for whatever reason, to convene today's sessions. How might you structure the last day of this MFT group? Why don't you have a go . . . you have seen what we practitioners have been up to over the past months . . . now it's your turn*'.

Chapter 6

Specific MFT activities

Why exercises, games and activities?

The many MFT activities, consisting of exercises and games, aim to address problematic interaction and communication patterns in a playful manner. They are a means to an end: To open up new experiences and different ways of viewing familiar dilemmas. A major aim is also the promotion of effective mentalizing, upregulating and down-regulating affect, so that group members are open to learning from different experiences and perspectives within a 'zone of tolerance' and creating a 'we' mode. The practitioners need to take responsibility for any mis-attunement, or indeed a total breakdown of mentalizing, as a result of having introduced a particular activity. In that event they need to show flexibility and create a better context to restore effective mentalizing. Although it is not ideal, it should also not be seen as a bad thing if, occasionally, mentalizing breaks down as a result of a playful activity being introduced. This is because every break in mentalizing provides an opportunity to notice what happened and repair the situation, a process which, in itself, provides an opportunity to strengthen the mentalizing capacity of the group. Which activities to choose depends on the issues and difficulties families present with and want or need to focus on, as well as on group processes. Choosing and adjusting MFT activities is never an easy task, as families' issues and needs not only vary but also because each MFT session has its own dynamics.

There are different ways in which MFT activities can be used, and much of this depends on their aims, how they are implemented and the feedback practitioners receive from families. A major *aim* of many of the activities and group activities is to help the group to coalesce and to become a kind of 'team'. Icebreaker activities in particular help to make the group a safe and creative context and to enable participants to have their anxiety levels reduced. Other activities focus on specific issues that families encounter in their daily lives, or the activity may focus on a particular symptom, disorder or problem. The time frame for each activity can vary, but, as a rule, it is between 10 to 30 minutes. The subsequent presentations and discussions can last anywhere from 20 to 60 minutes.

When it comes to the *implementation* of MFT activities, it is possible to stage whole group activities which involve everybody together: children, adolescents,

DOI: 10.4324/9781003442424-6

parents and other adults. Other activities can first be undertaken by each family on their own or with sub-groups (for example, parents and children), with their experiences and reflections being shared subsequently with the rest of the group. MFT activities can also be implemented individually, with everyone doing the task on their own. Another possibility is for children and parents to carry out an activity in parallel or together, and sometimes one or two families may do so in pairs, with the other families observing and reflecting. No matter how the activity is started, it is important that at some stage all families discuss their impressions or discoveries in the multi-family context, so that exchanges between *all* families can take place.

The way of asking for *feedback* from group members about MFT activities can also be varied. When each family is asked in turn to present to the rest of the group their work with a particular activity, the focus will be on this one family first, with the other families listening and then asking questions, as well as reflecting on what has been said and considering the implications for themselves and how they might tackle similar issues in their own families in the futures. Once the work with one family is completed, the practitioners can move on to the next family. Whilst this may seem to be a fair way of doing things, it also carries a risk of becoming repetitive and monotonous. To avoid this, one can begin with inviting two families to present their work to the whole group and then get each family to pair up with another one and interview each other about the results of the exercise. This is an easier task for families once they have observed how the practitioners have done this with the first two families. Practitioners can explain: '*You have observed how we talked about the activity with the Brown family and the Miller family. Now we could do the same with the four remaining families, but we suggest that you, Brown and Smith families, take over and that you each find one other family with whom you can find out about their work. The remaining families can join each family pair and assist them . . . so do this for the next 20 minute, that is, 10 minutes per family, and we can then talk about what really surprised you.*' Staged feedback can be also undertaken if a specific visual activity has been completed. The work can be displayed in the centre or the walls of the room and first be viewed by everyone simply walking around silently. One of the family members can then volunteer to present their display to all the other families, followed by small groups of families presenting their respective displays to each other and discussing these. Some activities have different phases, and this requires the practitioners to distinguish between these and focus the families' attention on each phase before moving on.

There is a seemingly infinite number of activities, and these are sub-divided, in alphabetical order, into three different categories. *Group activities* aim to help 'warm up' the therapeutic context and encourage participants to develop an interest in other families and their issues – and thus contribute to group cohesion and the development of a team spirit. The importance of strengthening relationships within the group should not be underestimated, as it is the group setting which provides the primary context for social learning and the 'we mode'. Following group activities can provide an opportunity to think about helpful links to, and implications for, life outside the group. *Family activities* focus on each (single) family temporarily and how they manage specific issues and tasks. Each family is then expected to share their experiences with the rest of the group or within a sub-group. *Problem-focused activities* deal with identifiable issues that tend to be related to a particular disorder or to a specific problematic interaction patterns. It is important for both family- and problem-based activities to include space for reflection and to think about transferring what has been learnt to the outside world. Some activities can be used for multiple purposes, for example, Speed Dating can be used to build group relations and to address specific problems. The activities described in this chapter have partly been developed or modified by ourselves, and many have been inspired by other clinicians and teams (see Schemmel et al., 2008; Asen & Scholz, 2010, 2017; Simic et al., 2023). We encourage readers to use them flexibly and to be creative in adapting and inventing activities that provide change contexts for the groups they run and to create opportunities for families to transfer what they have learnt to the home setting.

In order to make the activities more comprehensible, we describe them subsequently by providing the *instruction* in direct speech, just the way MFT practitioners might introduce them in a session. The instruction can of course be worded in very different ways, and the wording we list for each activity is only a suggestion. If it is delivered with a touch of theatricality, like with a loud and engaging voice and accompanied by appropriate body language, and sometimes with props (glasses, whitecoats, big pens), families are more likely to engage. By stating that '*we would like **you** to . . .*', the practitioners emphasize that the responsibility for making the activity 'happen' lies with the families. This allows the practitioners to observe what happens rather them remaining centrally involved. If group members are struggling with a task or are becoming dysregulated, the practitioners can provide a commentary on what they observe and then hand over to group members to manage the situation rather than jumping quickly themselves to the rescue. It is of course important that practitioners be mindful of any physical limitations or sensory issues group members may have and how these may impact their engagement in activities. Subsequently we also describe the *use* of each activity and how and under what circumstances it may be appropriate to employ it and how it could address specific issues. The *focus* tends to be developed during what has been referred to (in Chapter 3) as the 'third movement' of the 'systemic quartet': the reflection phase. We also note something specific for most of the activities, flagging issues practitioners may need to consider.

A. Group activities

Group activities have several functions: they are icebreakers, aimed at 'warming up' the therapeutic context and reducing any tensions, making the participants feel more at ease. Another aim of group activities is to further group collaboration and cohesion and thus allow families to feel safer, encouraging them to gradually begin to disclose difficulties and to feel open to learn from others. Finally, group activities provide opportunities for families to inadvertently learn from others as they observe their difficulties mirrored and potential solutions demonstrated by other families during the course of the activity. Practitioners may also observe interactions during a group activity which they decide to 'bookmark' and come back to at a later date.

Affect snapshots

Instruction

'During today's meeting, I'd like to take snapshots of each person here, including of myself. This of course requires your permission. Later we can look at the snapshots and guess what was on the mind of the person depicted.'
    Variation: *'Let's think of all the different types of feelings. Who can start us off? I am going to write a list. . . . I'd like each person here pick a feeling and then make a face showing that feeling. I will take a snapshot of each person. This of course requires your permission. Later we can look at the snapshots and guess the feeling each person depicted.'*

Use and focus

The focus is on guessing feelings or mental states of other group members and speculating on what can or might have triggered these. This activity involves group members having to pay close attention and mentalize one another. The emotional distance created by doing so via a photograph rather than by looking at individuals directly can be emotionally regulating and thus fosters more effective mentalizing. Group members can reflect on the limits of 'mind reading' and when and why one might one get it wrong.

Amoeba game

Instruction

'You probably have heard about Darwin's theory of species evolution. Let us look at it through a game, the amoeba game. In that game, there are five stages of evolution. First, the lowest stage is the amoeba stage. An amoeba is a simple cell which moves slowly by means of its flagella, never quite knowing where it goes (the practitioners mime this by using their arms in a swimming type of motion). *The second stage is the 'chicken phase'* (the practitioners mime chicken-like movements with their necks and elbows), *followed by the 'elephant stage'* (mimed*), next the 'monkey stage'* (mimed), *and the last, the final stage is becoming a human being. Only human beings have the privilege of sitting down on the chairs here but only once you have successfully climbed the Darwinian ladder. All group members now start in the amoeba stage, and when you meet another amoeba, you challenge it by playing "paper-scissors-stone", also known as "rock, paper, scissors"): you raise one*

hand in a fist and swing it down, say shoot and display again the symbol for one of these three objects. The person who wins the encounter morphs into the next Darwinian stage and becomes a chicken. And when a chicken meets another amoeba or chicken and wins, it morphs into an elephant – and so on. When you have done this, you find the next fellow player, be that an amoeba or any other animal. However, unlike Darwin's theory, if a chicken or even a monkey loses the encounter, they morph down, to the previous stage. So, at the end of the game, some of you will be humans; some elephants, monkeys or chickens; and some of you will be or even remain amoebas. So let us start: we are now all amoebas walking through the room and meeting other amoebas . . .'.

Use and focus

Can be used for all MFT projects at an early stage as an icebreaker activity. After freezing the interactions after a few minutes and asking everyone to remain in their respective 'animal' position, the practitioners can interview group members about their state of mind: '*What does it feel like still being an amoeba . . . and having been turned into a human, what might be advantages and disadvantages?*' Practitioners can focus on specific dynamics that occurred during the playful interactions and concentrate on themes such as: 'winning and losing', 'cheating', 'being human and no longer participating in the fun', 'feeling superior', 'feeling marginalized or denigrated'. At the end of the activity, group members can be invited to speculate: '*Why do you think we thought this was a good game to play at this point? Talk to each other for 2 minutes and then let's hear what everyone thinks!*'

Note: This game can be helpful as a way to engage more reserved parents in playful activity.

Animal families

Instruction

'*Imagine that you are all animals and that you all live peacefully together in a magic forest. What sort of animals might you want to be? Deer, elephants, moles, mice, birds, snakes, lions? Can each family decide for themselves what kind of animal family you want to be – or what you are going to do if each family member want to be a different animal? Please build a nest or other kind of home in this magic mountain. Then make a mask for yourself and one for your child to show what they would look like as that animal. . . . Once you have all done that, do make a family sculpt which shows how you are as a family now and how you would like to be in the future. Once all that has been done, each family will be invited to the middle to show both of their sculpts and explain to the rest of the group what that's been all about.*

Variation: '*Now there is a forest fire, how can the animal families help each other?*'

Use and focus

This activity suits families with young children, as well as adoptive or reconstituted families. Families need to mentalize themselves in order to decide on animal(s), including how they look to others and their characteristics. Families can be asked why they chose a particular animal. Further questions are: *'How did you feel as animal families? What was different from how things are usually? What would need to happen for you to become more like the sculpt they wish for? What happened when the forest fire broke out?'*

Note: Photos can be taken of each family sculpt and be referred back to when relevant at a later point in the group.

Anonymous letters

Instruction

'You have known each other for a few weeks now. Here is a piece of paper which contains all the names of the group members. We would like you to write behind each name, including your own name, one observation – and this could be praise, constructive criticism or some form of encouragement. It has to be something personal that you want to give him or her. Please change your handwriting so that nobody can recognize who the author of the anonymous letter is. Later we will read these anonymous letters out loud'.

Uses and focus

The activity can further build positive group relationships, as some people feel 'seen' by each others' observations. The focus can be on how people are experienced by others and whether anyone has received any surprising comments. Covert thoughts and feelings about others can be explored and the pros and cons of openness and transparency can be discussed. Practitioners can ask group members: *'What can one say openly, what can one only say anonymously? Why is this the case? What would need to be different for people to say openly what they think and feel about another person? Why is it important for criticism to be constructive, and why is it so difficult?'*

Blind trust

Instruction

'We want to play a game – it's about trust and who we can trust when and where. We have got a few blindfolds here and we want the parents to be blindfolded – so that they can really not see anything. And then we want their children to lead them through this room and perhaps even outside. Later we are going to make a pretend minefield

and then the children must be really careful to lead their parents through it. . . . There will be a third stage where the children will have to guide their parent through this minefield while describing the landscape of their choice.. . . . And then we want to turn the tables and the children are blindfolded and the parents lead them.'

Uses and focus

Being blindfolded can be dysregulating and thus impair effective mentalizing. It can also increase people's focus on their body and senses. The activity can be used to focus on establishing and questioning trust. Questions put to group members can include the following: *'Did you feel in good hands? When can one trust whom – and when not? Would one have found it easier to be led by someone from another family? What was most and what was least surprising? How does it feel to be responsible for someone who depends on one? How is it that mistrust grows – who knows about it?'* Links can be made to experiences and relationships outside of the group.

Body feelings

Instruction

'We cannot think of anyone who does not have feelings and emotions – even if we hide them from others or perhaps sometimes even from ourselves. And often we know what we feel, but not always where we feel it. So now we would like you to make a body outline of each person here, and for everyone to take it in turns and lie down on this wallpaper roll; then someone will draw the outline of your body. Each person will then get their picture and is requested to use different colours to draw in the feelings they have, put them wherever you think they 'live' – in your head, tummy, legs or wherever'.

Use and focus

Drawing and locating different emotions makes it easier for family members to become curious about feeling states. The focus can be on where certain feelings are located in their bodies in different individuals and how they manage hidden 'bad' feelings and enlarge 'good' feelings – and how interact with or influence each other.

Note: This activity can be preceded by getting group members to name typical feelings. These get written on a flipchart so that people carrying out the task can choose specific feelings.

Catch the ball

Instruction

'This ball here is going to be thrown from one person to another. Whoever catches it should say their name . . . that was a good round and now: whoever catches the ball should say one of their likes and one dislike (e.g., food, hobby, music etc) . . .

oh, well, we have learned a lot already, so in the next round whoever catches the ball should say two sentences about a member of their family . . . and the next round is just a memory test: whoever catches the ball should try and remember what the person who threw *the ball is called and what they have said about themselves and their family'*.

Use and focus

Best used in initial MFT meetings or when new families join with a view to building group cohesion, generating energy, raising affect and particularly engaging younger children.

Note: Issues can arise with the ball being thrown too hard or group members being excluded. The group should be encouraged to manage these issues themselves. Practitioners may choose to come back to specific issues at a later stage.

Circle game

Instruction

'Please place yourselves all in a big circle, with people joining hands and arms, not leaving a single gap. Look inside the circle. One of you, maybe you, Peter, comes out of the circle, and the circle is closing again. Peter, you need to find a way to get into this circle, right into the middle. Find a gap, or create one – try hard to get in there, any trick you want to use, but you must not hurt anybody.'

Variation: break out of the circle (one person is 'trapped' inside the circle and has to get out).

Use and focus

Best used in early phases of MFT and/or at a later stage if issues of exclusion and inclusion arise. Focus on how is it possible to 'fit in' or enter a circle of friends or a family: which tricks are permitted and which are not in order to enter the circle or escape from it? Group members can be asked to reflect on how it felt to be on the outside trying to get in or on the inside or having their entry blocked and how it felt to finally break through. It can promote effective mentalizing and be extended to topics and experiences relevant to families who feel marginalized or excluded.

Note: The game is more likely to succeed if a fairly resilient group member is first selected to try and enter or escape from the circle.

Conducting the multi-family orchestra

Instruction

'Sometimes we think that a group like this is a bit like an orchestra, in need of a conductor. Well, we do need a conductor now so that we can all harmonize with

each other. The good news is that we have a number of different conductors here who will do it all their own way.

We have here a few cardboard boxes that can provide the percussion; there are also glasses and a few musical instruments – it's up to the conductor to choose which are being used and what the music is like – and whether human voices or even a whole choir is needed. Later we can discuss what worked particularly well.'

Use and focus

The 'conductor' feels their agency valued as the whole group look to them for direction. 'We-ness' can be experienced in an embodied way through the sounds made. Different members can take it in turns to be in this position, and it can be a good opportunity to bring forward less engaged or less confident group members. The focus can be on experiencing collaboration, being clear about instructions and being able to play softly as well as loudly.

Duck, duck, goose

Instruction

'Thank you for everyone sitting in a circle. I am now walking on the outside of the circle, and as I go round, I will pat each person in turn on their shoulder and say 'duck'. At some point I will decide to say 'goose' instead of duck. At this point the 'goose' jumps up and has to race with me around the outside of the circle and try to sit in the spot they just vacated. Whoever gets there last takes over walking around the edge of the circle saying 'duck' until they decide to say 'goose' and there is another race. Let's try it!'.

Use and focus

This is a high-energy activity that can quickly raise the temperature in the room. It can be a good icebreaker at the beginning of the group, especially when younger children are in attendance. The group has to work together to manage keeping the arousal to a level that allows enjoyment of the activity. After the activity, if possible, there can be some reflections on what it was like, for example, to win or lose or be chosen or not be chosen to be a 'goose', all promoting the capacity for emotion regulation.

Fairy tale world

Instruction

'What type of person/character would you love to play? Create a costume and/or mask which represents this figure. Then introduce yourself briefly to the group in this new role. The group has then 45 minutes to invent a story or tale in which all the roles have a place. We will then produce the play. There are plenty of props,

from fancy dress(es) to paper, colouring pencils, face paint, glue, scissors and decorations'.

Use and focus

A suitable activity for families with young children. The group members have to work together over a short period of time to create a story. This pressure can raise arousal and makes negotiation a necessity. Dominant and quiet voices can be observed during the activity and, if appropriate, reflected upon after the activity. This activity supports families to experiment with new roles and behaviours in the 'as if' mode. Following the performance there can be an exploration of roles and ambitions, and families can also be asked how they can be their character for a day at home.

Note: Video recording of the performance can help families to later reflect on specific themes at a later stage. It can also be helpful to include the video as part of an ending ceremony.

Family excursions

Instruction

'We would like to do an outing with all of you next week. Let's talk about where we might go and what we might do . . . like the zoo, or a museum, or shopping centre . . . each family is responsible for the outing and their child(ren) . . . their care and safety . . . do bring enough money/food and make sure there is appropriate clothing'.

Use and focus

This activity is particularly useful for seemingly 'disorganized' and 'chaotic' families with pre-adolescent children. The group first needs to negotiate and decide on the details of the outing. This marks their agency. The focus can be on preparation and managing typical difficult or 'risk' situations as they emerge in natural circumstances. Practitioners are likely to notice many issues and interactions that they can 'bookmark' for later discussion. The activity can be followed by a video feedback session when families can view footage of the trip retrospectively and reflect, with some 'emotional distance', and thus be more capable of mentalizing.

Family meals

Instruction

'We would like you to think about a joint meal for everyone when we next meet. Can you do some planning together on how to make a joint meal – perhaps also food from different cultures? Food could also be bought together if we all go to a

supermarket.' On the day: *You have now one hour to prepare food, to eat it and then to clear up. We leave it entirely to you how you do this and how much you think your children should eat. Make the portions as healthy as you think they should be. We (staff) won't eat with you but we will be around to feed back our observation and any advice, if needed.'*

Use and focus

Families with eating issues/disorders and multi-problem families. The families first have to negotiate what to eat and to plan the meal. Leaving this process to them marks their agency. The focus is on the re-enactment of 'in vivo' crises around providing meals and eating. Themes of anxiety, control and authority often emerge. Families often feel reduced stigma and learn as they see other families struggle with similar issues to themselves.

Feeling fish

Instruction

'Today we want to introduce you all to fish and how they can feel. Well, it is arguable whether fish can feel anything, and therefore, to start with, we want each family member to draw a picture of a fish which shows something about how the family member feels a lot of the time. Here are a few example pictures, like this grumpy fish, a happy fish or this shy fish, and a scared fish, and here is a stressed fish. . . . We will now give each family some craft materials, and you will have 20 minutes to make a fish each. Parents can help their children if they are struggling – or perhaps it's the other way round? When you have finished your fish – and do take your time – please get up and show it to other group members and tell them about your fish and find out about their fish. And talk about why you made your fish look like it does.'

Variation: *A large 'sea scape' can be made with different features, including colourful choral, deep open water, dense reeds, dark caves, a whirlpool and so on. Families can be asked 'Where does your fish normally live? Can you use this Blu-Tac to stick it on the seascape?'*

Use and focus

Can be used with all families, including families with younger children. Locating the feelings in the fish rather than the person and focusing on the drawing task regulates affect and makes it easier for family members to move into talking about feeling states. Group members can be asked what sort of fish they are, and similarities and differences can be highlighted. They can also be asked: *'Were there any surprises? Would they like their fish or that of their family members to look different? What would it take for them to look that way?'* With the seascape, families are encouraged to find out about where the other members of their family placed their fish and whether there is any wish for change. If so, group members can be asked to talk to each other about how they might make that change happen.

Note: As a way of capturing change, a photograph can be taken of the seascape. Families can be asked to repeat the activity again at the end of MFT, and comparisons can then be made with the previous version.

Finding your place

Instruction

'If you look around and at each other you can see that we all look quite different. Some are tall and others are shorter. Why don't you form a line, defined by height. This means that the tallest person should be on the left end of the line and the smallest on the right end. Just line yourselves up and each person should place themselves where they think they fit.'

Next round: *'This time we want people to place themselves according to the colour of their hair: those with very black hair on the very left and those with white-blonde hair on the very right – and the rest should find their places somewhere between those poles.'*

Later – possibly: *'. . . and now place yourselves according to the colour of your skin . . .'*

Use and focus

Helping group members to look at each other properly and communicate about what they have in common and how they are different as well as fostering inter-personal collaboration. A variation of the activity involves asking group members to complete the activity but without talking. This increases the amount of attention everyone pays to the way each other look. Photos can be taken of the line-ups and then be shown to the group on a screen, inviting further discussions.

Frozen problems

Instruction

'Can each family think of a relationship problem that you have with your parents, partner, children or anyone else you are close to? If you had to turn this into a sculpture and then 'freeze' it, what might it look like? Choose a few group members to turn the problem into a frozen sculpture. We will take a quick snapshot of each sculpture so that we can all look at them afterwards.'

Later: *'While you are in this frozen position, we want to have some members of other families approach the frozen sculpture and walk around it to see it from different angles and make comments. What do you see happening? What does this evoke in you? What's going through everyone's minds?'*

Variation: *There can be a second 'round' of the activity where families make a sculpture which shows how they would like things to be.*

Use and focus

The process of making a frozen problem sculpture can highlight differences in family members' perspectives and key intra-family dynamics. Questions that arise include: *'Can problems be represented and read accurately? Is it possible to know how and what others feel? Why are similar problems being represented so differently?'* The activity provides families with an opportunity to have their difficulties 'seen' by the rest of the group, allowing for similarities and differences across families to be noted. Practitioners can extend the activity by asking: *'If one piece in the sculpture could be changed to improve the problem, which one might that be, and what would happen to the rest of the sculpture?'*

Geography sculpt

Instruction

'Let us all come to the middle of the room . . . this is where we are now (e.g., London, Paris, Berlin, New York), and this where north, south, east and west are. Now we want you each to go the area – the town, city, country – where you were born. If you were born in the place we are now, stay there, but if you were born somewhere else, do go there. . . . Find out from each other where all these places might be in relation to where you are now. Okay, you have done that now – gosh, some of you are here and some are over there . . . let us find out and go round. May I ask you, Jenny, where is it that you are standing right now? And who are you interested to find out more about – go and ask them, where are they?'

Later: *Now we want you to go where one of your parents was born . . . and now where the other one was born . . . and now where your grandparents were born.*

Later: *'It's now 20 years from now; imagine you can migrate where you want to . . . please go there and place yourself in the country and continent where you want to be'.*

Use and focus

Particularly useful when working with families from diverse cultural and geographic backgrounds. The focus can be on stories of migration, recent and to do with previous generations, as well exploring future aspirations. Families can be asked: *'So what would have to happen between now and then in order for you to be where you want to be 20 years from now?'* The activity can promote curiosity within and between families as well as identifying previously unknown connections. Group collaboration is required for the world to be mapped and for people to be able to identify their place.

Note: Younger children may find this activity difficult, and their own parents or other group members can be encouraged to help them.

Good-bye rituals

Instruction

'*Next time we meet it is the last time for the group (or for family B). How might you want to mark this? What would you all want to happen? Should there be a formal ceremony with speeches and certificates, or should it just be an informal celebration? Can you all think about this, and we leave it to you to organize the day . . .*'

Use and focus

It is left to the group to plan the whole event, including the practicalities, for example, around food or music, and to make decisions, for example, whether to issue certificates, and if so, who should do these. The family can enlist the help of the practitioners but only by assigning them appropriate tasks, such as providing some of the photos that have been taken over the course of the group or printing out the certificates. The focus of the activity can be on the advantages and disadvantages of celebrating an ending, and the activity can bring forth different stories, traditions and rituals of endings gone by. The activity can also bring with it a sense of achievement as the group mark their time together in a way that feels good to them.

How it all started . . .

Instruction

'*Can the parents please make a circle facing each other and the children remain seated in the outside circle. We are now asking the parents to, with our help, explain how it all started, the difficulties or problems that brought you here. You have about 3 minutes each. Explain how it changed family life and maybe also your relationships with friends and others. When you have finished, we will ask the children to come into the circle in the middle and for you to listen to their conversation.*'

Use and focus

Can be done at the beginning of MFT to help group members to discover similarities and connect people with one another. Curiosity is provoked first in the children and then in the parents as they are invited to 'listen in' to the conversation. The structure of the activity and the fact that the observing group is not expected to give any responses can make individuals more available to then hear what the reflecting group has to say. Differences between the children's and the adult's accounts are common. It can be useful to highlight this and to ask the group to think about why this may be the case, as a way of stimulating mentalizing.

Note: Some family members can use the space to be critical of one another. Practitioners need to judge the extent to which this may be having a negative impact and, if so, consider whether to pause the conversation then and there – or to 'bookmark' it and to come back to it after the activity.

How others see you

Instruction

'*Here are a few Post-Its for everyone. Can you please write on them four adjectives, positive and negative, you think that other group members here might use to describe you. Write these down and stick the Post-Its on you and meet others and check out what they make of your self-descriptions. And then write one adjective about that person on a Post-It and stick it on their back. And later you can compare the different descriptions.*'

Variation: '*Can you write on a Post-It Note four adjectives, positive and negative, that correspond to how people who know you would describe you? Write them down and stick the Post-It on yourself, then meet others and discuss what they think of your descriptions. Then write on another Post-It Note an adjective about yourself that you think others don't see, know or recognize. Then you can compare the different descriptions.*'

Use and focus

This is particularly suitable for families with adolescents and adults. It requires mentalizing of both the self and others. After the activity, group members can be asked whether there were any surprises. There can be a focus on speculating as to why the self-ascribed adjectives may be similar to, or different from, those the other group members had posted. Group members can be asked '*What do you think is it that gives people the impression that you are . . . ?*' A discussion can be had about whether people want their hidden characteristics to be discovered and recognized or remain hidden. What might be for and what against it? Links can be made to issues to do with identity development, how people present themselves outside of the group and what that might be about.

Labelling oneself

Instruction

'*People here are new; they haven't met before. Could each of you write five words (or drawings) on this little sticker which say something about you as a person and then stick it on? You can then walk around in this room and look at what people have said about themselves – and ask questions if you like.*'

Variation: '*Write down first impressions others have of you (correct or not) – what is it that you do that gives people the impression that you are . . . ?*'

Use and focus

This is suitable for most families. This activity requires mentalizing of self and others and can be good for group cohesion, as it promotes curiosity and can quickly lead to the identification of non-problem related similarities. There can be a focus on the accuracy – or otherwise – of the different labels.

Note: Younger children may find this game difficult, but they can be involved by reducing the number of adjectives required and/or by using pictures instead of words.

Lie detector

Instruction

'It may be difficult for some of you to tell lies, but here is a game you might enjoy – guessing what's true and what may be a lie. Can each of you take four Post-It Notes and write on them three things that are true about you and one statement that is a lie. Put these on your chest or head and walk around the room. Be a little detective and meet all other group members, one by one, and guess their lie. See whether you can get it right the first time around and not the fourth time. Don't make your own lie easy.'

Use and focus

This activity can be used in the first or second MFT session to generate energy and for people to meet one another. The focus is on how good or bad one can be at guessing – and at mentalizing others. Questions put to group members include the following: *'What are the give-away signs to look out for? Was it more difficult to formulate the lies or the true statements? Are there occasions when it is necessary to lie – and are there 'good' lies? What does it feel like to lie and what does it feel like to be lied to?'*

Note: Younger children may need help with this, and group members need to be encouraged to provide appropriate support.

'Live' sculpting

Instruction

'Please come with me, John: you have a unique chance now to sculpt your family – your parents, siblings and other important and relevant persons. You can move them as if they were made out of plasticine or rubber. They will move the way you want them to, but they cannot talk. Find a typical position and posture for each of them. If some of your family members are not here and you think they are important, you can pick use persons from other families to stand in.' The practitioners surround the sculpt area with a red rope which is meant to signify the 'problem

area' and explains this. '*Now find a place and posture for yourself in this sculpt. And now I would like all of you to be silent for 2 minutes and feel the situation. Afterwards I would like you to come out of the sculpt again and someone else from the group here can take your position . . . so what does it feel like in there – and what does it look like from the outside? Why is this person in that position?' If you want to take someone form the family out of the sculpt – do so and replace him or her with someone form the group. Sometimes people find it helpful to look at themselves and their family from the outside'.* Later the practitioners will ask the family to leave the sculpt, and the red rope remains in its place. They place a green rope near a window and ask the sculptor: '*Was there a time when you felt good as a family? Maybe during a holiday, when celebrating something or when you played a game or had an outing? Please sculpt now a situation when you and the family all felt well. Place your family here, surrounded by the green rope. . . . Please all remain in that position for 2 minutes without saying anything'.* The observing group will be asked to comment and share observations and their own experiences. After this the practitioners can say: '*Well, that sounds all pretty good but sadly you as a family are these days in a different place . . . but what would need to change so that you could all move in the direction of the green circle?*'

Use and focus

The focus is on visually representing problems and to get group members to 'feel' each family's position. Lesser heard family members can be given agency if they are the ones requested to make the sculpts. New ideas and perspectives about how families may have got 'stuck' and might experiment with taking new positions are generated, and families can be asked how they might take some of the ideas home.

Note: 'Live sculpting' is a powerful tool for a collaborative way of working when other families are asked to move around a family's sculpture and speculate on the mental states of the figures. The members of the sculpted family can then be asked about the comments and whether there is anything they would like to change about what has been said about their situation. The other members of the group then get together to think about changes to the sculpture that might meet the family's expectations. The group then appoints a sculptor who modifies the family sculpture according to what the group has suggested. The family holds the new pose. Further speculations about the mental states of each figure are invited.

Lost property

Instruction

'*You don't really know each other, so we want you to move around the room and meet someone. You tell them your name, they tell you theirs, and you give them one of your items – important or not – and they give you theirs in return. Then you move on and meet a new person, to whom you give the first person's object and name, and they do the same with the object in their possession. You continue until someone says stop, at which point you have to find the person whose object you are holding and talk to them'.*

Use and focus

This can be used with all families to build group cohesion. Families can be encouraged to use the feelings evoked by the task to address themes around building trust – and related fears. Links can be made to similar situations outside of the group and how these have been managed. Differences and similarities can be highlighted as a way of opening new perspectives and possibilities.

Note: This exercise can lead to family members talking about reasons why they have come to be mistrustful of others as a result of being mistreated, for example, having experienced abuse, neglect, racism or other forms of oppression. Practitioners may then get the parents and other adults to consider whether or not it is appropriate for children to be exposed to such accounts.

Masked ball

Instruction

'This is an activity just for the adolescents in this room. Let us imagine that it is the year 2085 and all the young persons here are alive and old. You haven't seen each other for more than half a century, and someone smart got all your new addresses and has arranged an improvised tea party. Do come and sit around this table with coffee, tea and cakes, and you can all make up your own stories of your lives – the more imaginative and the wilder, the better. This is why I have brought these (Edwardian) masks; they are bit strange, but they will help you when you put them on, as you are no longer this person sitting here but someone quite different, and it will help you to catapult yourself into the future . . . now that you have your masks on and you see all your colleagues looking so different, we can start the fantasy game . . . so let us start, I am putting a mask on, too. . . . We have not seen each other for such a long time, I have literally forgotten your names – what are your full names now? How many children and grandchildren do you have now? And in your case, how many marriages and divorces have you had? Do you still suffer from an eating disorder/ADHD/depression? Did you ever go to university, or did you end up in Hollywood right away? Start to talk to each other and find out where you have got to . . .'

Use and focus

This activity is best used towards the end of MFT work with families containing adolescents. The playfulness of the activity and the fact they are talking from behind a mask frees them up to think outside of their current situation. Quite often the stories adolescents make up arc hopeful. The focus can be on thinking about hypothetical futures from which group members can view their current lives retrospectively. Questions that can be put to the adolescents include the following: *'When you look back on your life, what was/were the turning point(s)? What do you imagine your parents make of what they have heard?'* The adolescents can later ask what their parents actually thought about what they heard, and a conversation can be had about how different trajectories can be supported or averted.

Medieval kingdom

Instruction

'Imagine you live in a kingdom, far, far away. Please decide who lives in your kingdom – like king, queen, prince, princess, maid, servant, fool, knight, peasant, craftsman, merchant, jailer and so on. Once you have decided who is who, please find ways of dressing up – you can make hats, crowns, jewellery, tools – whatever you like. There are a lot of props here; just have a look. Then make a kingdom where everything works out well. And we would like everyone here to be part of the kingdom'.

Variation: *'Let's imagine there is a revolution against royalty! What happens next?'*

Use and focus

This activity is popular with families containing pre-adolescent children. The focus is on role choices, negotiations and collaboration. Families get an experience of interacting harmoniously in a world where everything works out. Later they can be asked how this felt and, if there was a revolution, how this might affect their feelings, needs and plans. Group members can also be asked whether the activity reminded them of anything at home.

Photo stories

Instruction

'Between now and next time we meet, please select seven photographs that explain the history of your family, just seven of the most important photos. This will mean deselecting a few. Next time we would like to see and hear the story of your family or of family life'

Variation: *Each family member chooses two or three photographs.*

Use and focus

The process of selecting the photographs requires families to discuss key events and decide which ones are most important to include. They can later be asked: *'Who did the choosing? Which photos were deliberately excluded? Which memories are evoked, and which good stories come to mind?'* The sharing of photos can promote group curiosity and improve connections as families find out more about one another.

Popping balloons

Instruction

'We would like for each family to sit together, and we will give you Post-It Notes with each family's surname on it – including your own. We want you then to write down three positive statements about each family. Once you have done so, we will gather up the statements and place them in a balloon for each family, then blow the balloon up and write the family name on it. And later each balloon will be popped, with the statements floating down to the floor, and each family can then see what has been written about them'.

Use and focus

This is a variation of Anonymous Letters, except the balloons contain positive statements only. The focus can be on validation of families' strengths. What did they particularly like to hear? There can be further conversation about how these strengths can continue to be seen by others once the group has finished. The 'pop' of the balloon provides a sense of excited anticipation and punctuates the move from one family to the next.

Protect your mum

Instruction

'We think a lot of children here react strongly when someone threatens their mum, but sometimes these very same children can be quite aggressive towards their own mum. In this game, the children team up with their mums. They have to stand in front of her to protect her. Here's a soft ball, and the aim is for one mum to hit another mum with the ball on the part of her body that her child is protecting. The mother-child team can move around, but be careful not to get lost! Here we go!'

Use and focus

Good exercise for or poorly structured families and families with defiant children. The focus could be on *'What is real protection actually? When and from whom did you ever need protection? What sort of protection do you need? Why do we sometimes think that other people can't defend themselves on their own?'*

Remote control

Instruction

'Wouldn't it be wonderful when we use a remote control and – bang – the TV or DVD works. Just a push of the button and there is a sudden change. If only this was

possible in real life; it would simplify many things and then parents could get their children to do exactly as they want. And perhaps the children could do the same with their parents. Or the other way round. Just by pressing a button, mum jumps up and does what her little darling son wants her to. Or mum presses a button, and the children do exactly as they are told. Well, we have good news for you: we have invented just that type of remote control. Here is one for each family, try for yourself – point it at me and tell me what you want me to do . . . (practitioners hand the child a remote control and then does exactly as the child tells him to do). *Who here wants to have a go and see how it works in your family? Who here wants to be remote controlled by their child?'*

Later: *'Can we now have a group with the parents and another with just the children, and each group makes a remote control with just the most important five buttons to improve family life – and we can compare these later.'*

Use and focus

Families containing children with behavioural issues. The focus can be on what is needed to get control over children and adults. The following questions can be put to group members: *'How and when might remote controls be handy? How is it possible to control others without an actual remote control? Who should be controlling whom? What is too much and too little control? Does self-control come into this? What are the differences and similarities between the buttons chosen by the children and the parents?'* Each family is encouraged to consider building their very own three-button remote control which can be employed between sessions, with feedback provided during the next MFT meeting.

Responsibility and irresponsibility boxes

Instruction

'Most people feel responsible in certain situations and for certain people. But sometimes we act irresponsibly. We would like each person in the room to think of three examples of acting responsibly and one or two examples of acting irresponsibly. Place these statements in one of these two boxes. When everyone has done so, we will pick out a few of these statements from both boxes and read them out loud, anonymously, so that nobody will know who has written the note – only the author of the note. We can then discuss your views.'

Use and focus

Curiosity is naturally stimulated, as people will be trying to guess who wrote what. Discussions can focus on the different views as to what is responsible and what is not. The protection of anonymity allows people to share perspectives that they may not voice otherwise, and agency can be promoted by asking the group members to think about how they might act in a responsible way between now and next time. They will be asked to share their experiences only if they want to.

Riskometer

Instruction

'It's difficult for most parents to know how much autonomy their young person should have, especially when it comes to them making difficult decisions. But parents are often held back by fears, whether well-founded or not, and that may make it difficult to let the young person to move forward on their own. Here is a sheet of paper for each parent. Scale it vertically from 0 to 5, with 0 meaning that you don't let your teenager take any risks and that you take care of everything and supervise them most of the time and 5 meaning that you let the young person manage every-day matters and responsibilities totally by themselves. Put each of your young person's everyday living tasks (e.g., personal hygiene, taking medication, waking up in the morning, getting to school/college on time, etc.) on the riskometer and write down the level of risk you are currently taking on all these tasks and responsibilities for your young person. Then compare your results, first in separate groups of mothers and fathers and then as a parental couple.'

Use and focus

This activity is useful for families with older teenagers and young adults. The discussion between parents can focus on how to guide a young person towards autonomy: *'Should one just wait for them to become autonomous, or should one let go of areas of responsibility to help them become autonomous? What risks is one prepared to take? How can one reconcile the differences between parents' points of view?'*

Shells and balloons

Instruction

'Sometimes we hang onto things when we should really throw them away. Try telling that to a hoarder . . . but it's not just things we hang onto; it can be feelings, new discoveries and also grievances. Here are two pieces of paper for everyone, one white and one red, and everyone gets one little shell and one balloon. Now we want each of you to think of one thing you want to hold onto from what happened in the group and to you today until the next time – and one you want to let go. It could be a problem, a discovery, a feeling, a thought, whatever . . . write down the thing you want to hold onto on the white piece of paper and put the shell next to it, and then write down what you want to get rid of on the red piece of paper and place the balloon next to it. And here is the homework: over the next week on each even day,

put the shell in your pocket or bag and hold onto what you learned this time. And on each uneven day, put the balloon in your pocket/bag – and let go of it. Next time we can talk about it if you wish'.

Use and focus

The focus can be on self-mentalizing and developing agency as one is given the choice between holding on and letting go. Possible questions put are: *'Is this sometimes difficult to do? When are those times? What makes it easier/harder?'* The intersession task supports the transfer of learning outside of the session.

Smoke signals

Instruction

'Who can explain what a smoke signal is? Well, that's what we believe the Native Americans did in the Wild West. . . . But here it's a bit different . . . we can make a sound, a song, a beat or a physical movement. Who would like to show their 'smoke signal'? Any person in the group here can pick up the smoke signal someone else makes by copying it as best they can. They then make their own smoke signal for another member to pick up and so on'.

   Variation – Miming Chinese whispers.

   'We would like to divide you into groups of about six persons and form lines with their backs to each other. The first person in each line turns around and reads silently at a sentence written by a practitioner (for example: 'I'd like us to spend more time together' or 'I'd like you to be proud of what I do'). She then turns to the other person, taps them on the back to make them turn round, mimes the message, then the second person turns to the third and so on. At the end, everyone says what they understood'.

Use and focus

This can be used for all families that struggle with of miscommunication, vulnerability and attachment problems. With signals not being heard, being misunderstood, being too complicated or being too quiet, it is hard to respond. The activity focuses attention by demanding that the group members pay close attention to one another. Afterwards they can explore how sometimes it can feel too risky to put a signal out in case someone doesn't see it or gets it wrong or one puts out an extra loud signal in order to make sure one does get heard. Questions for group participants: *'What does it feel like to wait for someone to pick up your signal or not to have your signal picked up at all or for someone to get it wrong? What does it feel like to get it wrong? What are the reasons for getting it wrong?'* Links can be made to typical interactions between children and parents at home and how misunderstandings do happen.

Note: It may be beneficial to make some additional 'parent-only' time following this activity, particularly when younger children are involved, as it is not always appropriate for parents to be transparent about their responses to their children's attachment behaviour in their presence.

Spaghetti and marshmallows

Instruction

'Families do have structures – even if these are invisible, unlike architectural structures like towers and other high-rise buildings. But invisible family structures can become visible when we observe how family members relate around a specific task. This one is important because it allows family members to remain connected to each other and experiment with support. Structure must be strong and stable, in order not to fall and drag individuals down with it. But that structure must also be sufficiently flexible to enable adaptation to the necessary evolution of individuals and family. So, you'll find on your table some dry spaghetti and some marshmallows. Each family has to make a structure or building out of these two ingredients. It can be high or low, and it has to represent what you think you are like as a family. But remember, one has to be careful when working with dry spaghetti, it breaks easily – and as far as marshmallows are concerned, the more you eat, the less stable will be the foundations of your building. It's important that you work together as a team! Let's go! You have 15 minutes!'

Use and focus

This is a suitable activity particularly for poorly or rigidly structured families. It allows them to explore family structures in playful and (initially) non-verbal ways. One focus is on family cooperation and the allocation of roles. Group members are also invited to make comments about the thoughts and feelings the work invokes in them and link them to their family of origin and current family.

Note: Family structure is a rather abstract concept and may be difficult for younger children to grasp. Parents will need to tune into their child to make the task relevant to them, keeping them engaged and preventing them from eating all the marshmallows! This activity tends to provoke competition between families as to which has done the 'best' structure.

Speed-dating

Instruction

'Can people form two circles please, one which looks outwards and, opposite it, looking inward – so that each person is opposite another person? Can all the people sitting in the inner circle interview the one sitting opposite them about what food they like on each other about your likes and dislikes. You have only 2 minutes each to find this out, and then when we ring the bell, the adults have to move one

seat to the left – and then you do the same thing again. And later it will get faster and faster . . . you'll get quite breathless.'

Use and focus

Can be done at the beginning of any MFT session as an icebreaker and with a view to connecting families or later on to help families focus their thinking on a particular issue. It can be used to generate energy, but at the same time the knowledge that people will 'move on' quickly makes connecting with others a less anxiety-provoking task. It can also be used to help focus family members' attention on the issues that have brought them to participate in MFT.

Note: Each time group members move around one place, the time they are given to talk to the person opposite them gets shorter – until they are answering the same question in only 5 or 10 seconds. Questions can be about *'what happened in school yesterday'* or *'at home last night'*, about *'the problems that brought each family to the group'* or about *'one wish that they would want to come true'*. Alternatively, the activity can be used to promote reflection in the form of *slow speed dating*, with longer time spans for each person to talk and listen, up to 2–5 minutes. When the activity has finished, the whole group can be invited by the practitioners: *'Can someone please share with the group something really surprising that they heard during the activity?'*

Stepping into someone else's shoes

Instruction

'Can you all sit in a circle? Put a piece of paper under your feet and draw the contours of your shoes. Now get up and move to the left and stand in the shoeprints of your neighbour. Imagine you are that person now and continue the discussion you just had.'

Variation: *'Imagine you are that person. Now I am going to come and ask the person you are a question. Let me see, you are Charlie, is that right? (a father in his son's shoes). Now, tell me, Charlie, why do you think children sometimes don't like to go to school? . . . OK, Charlie, now it is your turn; choose someone to ask a question. Remember to address them as the person they are being rather than the person they are.'*

Use and focus

This can be used for any family. The focus is on perspective change and on whether it helps to better understand where other people are coming from. Family members are often surprised at how well other people do in their shoes, and in this way mentalizing is stimulated.

Note: The variation can work well with younger children or when the practitioners want to focus the group's attention on a specific theme or issue.

Stranded on an island

Instruction

'Imagine you are all on a cruise on this wonderful ocean liner. All is comfortable, you enjoy life . . . there are no worries . . . but suddenly the boat hits a rock and the boat sinks – everyone has to jump ship and use the life boat, which cannot take everybody – what are you going to do? And when you arrive on the island, there is nobody. Captain and board personnel remain on the sinking ship, so the families have to help themselves. What do you do when you arrive on the island. How are you going to survive? Please find ways of making a script together and play these situations'.

Use and focus

Families of all ages can participate in this activity. The high affect and need for collaboration mean that this activity works best in the more advanced stages of group work. The focus can be on families' ability to plan, organize, collaborate and allocate appropriate roles. The focus can also be on who the leaders were and who struggled to make their voice heard. Families can be asked whether they saw any particular strengths or skills in anyone, and they can be encouraged to think about how the explored survival skills can be used to manage their everyday lives.

Stringing along

Instruction

'Here are a few ropes (or strings), and we want you to use them to show how close and distant you are from each other. It may be the case that you each see this differently, and that's why we would like each family member to do their own version. You hold one end of the rope and please give the other end of the rope to another family member, maybe the one that you think is least close to you . . . and now place the rest of your family somewhere along the rope, the way you see family relationships – they don't have to be all in a straight line. They may not agree – it's just the way you see it. Later everyone will have their turn and we can take a few pictures so that we can remember how people did it and then talk about it'.

Use and focus

The focus is on visualizing the respective distance and closeness between family members. There can be discussions on what is culturally appropriate or not and how distance and closeness can be spoken about and changed if it is felt necessary. Families may be asked to think about what changes might need to take place at home for the desired changes to be achieved and be given the option to report back to the group next week.

Surprise birthday party

Instruction

'Imagine you have just found out that it is X's birthday today (pointing at one child)*. You are all here and want to give X a birthday party. How do you go about it? Please plan a party during the next 15 minutes – and then give it. X, you are not allowed to hear anything about it, so you have to sit/play with us for that time in another room.'*

Use and focus

Suitable for families with young children. Group members will have different ideas about what a 'good' birthday party looks like. The focus can be on children's expectations and likely frustrations – and the importance, or otherwise, of presents. The focus can also be on giving and receiving and gratitude. This can be explored with the question: *'Have you ever had someone not recognize the value of what you've done for them?'*

Talent show

Instruction

'We would like the children to go to another room and make a talent show for the parents, like the X Factor. There will be no winner but just a chance for them to show the group something they enjoy. Children can show their talents; it can be anything from singing or dancing to gymnastics or athletics, TikTok dances, football tricks, a talk on their favourite subject – whatever. Today we think about what everyone can do, and next time we finish rehearsals before the actual performance. Think about any props or accessories you might want to bring from home for your performance.'

Use and focus

This activity promotes children's sense of self and agency. It celebrates their strengths, and it allows the focus to be on something positive. Following the children's performances, parents can to think about what makes them proud of their children, and group members can reflect on how their strengths could become more evident in day-to-day life.

Note: With the parents' permission, the practitioners can take photos of each child's performance and share these as part of the goodbye ceremony. This activity works best when there is a separate room for the children to prepare their performances.

Tower of Babble

Instruction

'We have a lot of families here from all over the world, so there are many different languages and it is really difficult for people to understand each other. We would like everyone to get up and pretend to speak some ancient or utterly incomprehensible fantasy language, to meet other people in the room, to make yourselves understood and begin to have a conversation and do something together and then move onto the next person. You can use your hands and arms to support the language and make yourself understood. And when you have spent 1 minute or so talking with that person, then move onto the next person.'

Later: *'Now we need some pretend interpreters who are really good at guessing what has been said. Can you listen to what two people are saying and translate it into English, and the two people can non-verbally signal whether this translation is correct or not?'*

Use and focus

This activity can be used when many different languages are spoken in a group and when some families from different cultures are at risk of getting marginalized. The instruction can be translated into the relevant minority language via an audio translation app. The focus can be on what can be communicated by other means than language and how one gets marginalized and misunderstood. This can be related to scenarios both inside and outside the group setting.

Tug of war

Instruction

'We notice that the children are getting more and more restless. How about using any surplus energy and converting it into action? How about playing tug of war? Let's form two teams – maybe first all the children on one side and the parents on the other. Who knows who is going to win? Later you can also mix the teams and pick a few children for the parents' team – and a few parents for the children's team. We also need a referee – who is going to volunteer? The referee can explain the rules and make sure people stick to it. And we will have a few rounds'.

Use and focus

Best used with families with pre-adolescent children. The focus can be on winning and losing and whether one should let the weaker ones win. What is fun and when do things get serious – is there an overlap? Families can reflect on who the strongest team is and why, who felt close to whom during the game and what experiences people have of working as teams. Links can be made to similar experiences outside of the group.

Wellness farm

Instruction

'*You have all worked very hard today – wouldn't it be good to take a rest and be pampered? Have you ever been to a health farm? We certainly haven't – much too expensive and time consuming! The good news is that we have a health farm here. All we need is a bit of imagination. . . . Let's imagine that half of you are clients and the other half are staff. We'll give everyone a number, 1 and 2. . . . And all the 1s are staff and all the 2s are clients. The clients have to arrange their chairs in a circle facing inwards – and the staff take their position behind the client – one person behind each chair. You are the 'feel good worker'. For 3 minutes it is your job to make you client relax and recover their energy. You can use your hands and massage – but only if your client allows you to. Or you can talk or even sing to them to make them feel good. You might use music or whatever. But it is important that your client like what you do – otherwise they can't feel good. After 3 minutes you move onto the next client.*'

Possible part 2: '*We are going to ask you to rank the feel-good workers in the order you think they came. We'll compare it with reality*'.

Use and focus

This activity is best used during the later stages of MFT. The activity builds trust, as the 'helped' person is in a relatively vulnerable position. The helper has to mentalize the person they are helping and use feedback in order to adapt their behaviour. Afterwards they can be asked: '*How did you know what to do? How did you know when the person was enjoying it or not enjoying it? What did it feel like to help/to be helped?*' The activity provides an opportunity to practice empathy, express and respond to needs and validate help. It also highlights individual differences of what people find helpful and relaxing. Links can be made to being in a helper and helped situation outside of the group as well as how and why people can become 'self-helpers'.

Who has ever . . . ?

Instruction

'*Let's form a large circle. I'm going to ask a question to everybody, and whoever feels addressed has got to go for a few seconds to the space in the middle of the circle and shout 'I did!' and clap their hands. So let us start: Who's ever got a really bad result in maths? Who's ever pushed his brother or sister? Who's ever been excluded from the classroom? Who has ever managed to make their parent laugh when they scolded them? Who has ever been bullied?'*

Use and focus

Can be used at any point, but most often at the beginning as family members are getting to know one another. Can also be used to highlight common experiences and to put group members at some ease before a new or difficult topic us tackled. Highlighting common experiences improves group cohesion, particularly when some group members feel marginalized or stigmatized. By physically stepping into the middle of the circle, these commonalities are amplified. There can be a focus on a number of themes and related feelings, like shame and courage, exclusion and inclusion.

   Note: Some family members may not participate, choosing not to disclose certain experiences. The practitioners could indirectly address this by wondering aloud: *'Do you think everyone here feels brave enough to move into the middle? Some people might feel a bit too embarrassed to do it. That is quite normal. I wonder what you could do to make sure everyone feels safe to step forwards'*.

Wink murder

Instruction

'We first need someone who wants to be a detective – who would like to be the detective? Okay, there is going to be a murder in this room; don't worry, it's just a game – and you need to work out who the killer is. You need to leave the room now so that the murder can happen, and we will call you back in once that's happened. Can you families here decide who the murderer is – any volunteers? Okay, that's settled, dear murderer. You kill people in this room by winking at them. If a group member is being winked at, they have to pretend to die. The more dramatic, the better, like this . . . ahhh . . . ooooooh . . . When the detective comes back into the room, they have to guess who the murderer is. But an adult detective only gets one guess. Children get three guesses'.

Use and focus

This activity is suitable for all families, especially those with children between 5 and 12 years of age. It can be useful activity to integrate latecomers. The activity involves the group working together and closely attending to each other, 'hiding' one's feelings and intentions, attempting to read facial cues and managing anticipation. In subsequent discussion, the themes of being excluded and included are focused upon. Questions that can be raised are: *'When is it useful to be disloyal to one's group? What is it like to witness someone in a difficult position?'*

Wrong-hand writing

Instruction

Part 1 *'Today we are going to do something strange. You will all get paper and pens, and we are going to dictate a text that we want you to write down, not with your writing hand (usually the right) but with the non-writing hand. Please start writing: 'Today I decided to write with my other hand. I really appreciate this effort, which allows me to push myself. I think I'll keep doing it for the rest of the day or even the rest of my life'. When you have written this, please mark your effort just like a teacher, from 1 to 5, with 1 being excellent and 5 being awful. we are then going to collect all the specimen writing and will place it before a panel – who would like to volunteer? We need five people. So, let us have a look at this specimen: panel, what grade do you give it? Would the author like to say how they rated their own writing?'*

Part 2 *'we would like you to now form sub-groups of three; we can do this at random: 1,2,3,4,5: all the 1s in this part of the room, all the 2s in that part of the room . . . etc. Take 30 seconds to decide who is going to be the writer with the wrong hand. We would like them to write the text of their choice, and we want the other members of the small group to help the writer to succeed in their project. Can the writers explain how they want to be helped or not . . . now start.'*

Use and focus

This is a useful activity for families with adolescents or adults. The focus can be on efforts to do something that is not natural and on helping someone who makes the effort to do something that is not natural. Questions put to group members include: *'How do you assess yourself? What criteria do you use to assess yourself and others? Why is it different or similar? What are ingredients of good or bad help? Who was excluded or overinvolved and why?'* Links can be made to situations when one has had to step outside of one's comfort zone and yet manages to be successful.

B. Family activities

The activities presented in this section address intra-family issues and relationship problems. They aim to identify family strengths as well as to make overt otherwise hidden thoughts, feelings and values. Families need to know other families a little bit before embarking on some of the activities in this section, as they concern personal issues. Many of these activities will be undertaken first in single-family settings and then presented to other members of the group. Most whole-group activities can also be used to identify and address intra-family dynamics, though this is often done by 'bookmarking' and returning to them later either with the whole group or, more often, with individual families or sub-groups.

Care tags

Instruction

'*Who knows what a care tag is? Think of items of clothing or fabrics and the washing symbols and instructions on them, which may say 'delicate', 'wash hot', 'hand wash' or 'do not iron'. Let's get away from the actual washing and think about what care tags you would want to be attached to you and for managing your emotions, like when you feel anxious, sad or angry. Now can each group member make a care tag that describes how you would feel most cared for? Here are some empty care tags for everyone, and you can write on those.*'

Use and focus

The activity requires the labelling of emotions, and everyone has to mentalize themselves, including thinking about their needs and how they regulate their feelings. Questions put to family members include: '*How accurately can they do this? Do they need any help with the task? Can they make their needs known? If not, why might this be? Whose role is it to care for whom, and how can others outside of the group be made aware of each person's care instructions?* ' This activity can also be elaborated upon in Slow Speed-Dating.

Clay family sculptures

Instruction

Part 1: '*We would like each person/family to use the clay to make a sculpture of your family as you see it now. Make all the members of the family and place them on the wooden board. Make them as big or small as you like or how important they seem to you. Pay attention on how they are positioned in relation to each other. This can have something to do with their problems or illness or just how you experience it. And give your sculpture a name or title. You have 30 minutes to complete the task – and afterwards we pretend that we are in a modern art gallery and each person presents their work to the others*'.

Part 2: '*We would like the artists now to lean back and listen to the experts on family sculptures. We would like you to pretend that this is your job – an art critic – and that you have to describe and perhaps interpret the sculpture. What are your ideas as to who is in this sculpt and what it all means?* '

Use and focus

Differences in family members' perspectives on the problem and key intrafamily dynamics are highlighted. Similar questions as those listed in the Live Sculptures activity can be put to families, like: '*If something had to change in this family – where would one start? Where might one place the illness/problem? What would the family look like if the problem/illness was no longer there? Where should something change – who is most and least interested in promoting it? Which of the many relationships might one want to change first? And if one moved that person closer to that one – what would happen to the others?'*

Conflict maps

Instruction

'Can each family draw the floor plan of your flat/house? Mark in red where the typical battles/fights/arguments take place. Also do a map of your area, where you are, the neighbours, shops, school and so on. Also mark where the most problematic behaviours occur.'

Use and focus

This activity lends itself to the work with high-conflict families. The focus can be on discovering the concrete links between context and problematic interactions and then identifying ways of avoiding confrontations in the future. Questions: *'How do you explain that your teenage children have most of their arguments outside the bathroom? If you all wanted to reduce these, what would need to happen at home? How come you and your husband always argue in the bedroom? What would happen if each time you are tempted to have yet another argument, you change the 'scene of the crime' by pausing and moving into another room before continuing to argue? Would a change of 'crime scene' really help? What else could reduce the conflict?'* The focus of attention on the map rather than each other helps families to have conversations about conflict in a more regulated way. Following these conversations, family members can be invited to think about one change they might make at home as a way of trying to reduce conflict and to report back to the group as to whether it was effective next time.

Dream house

Instruction

'We would like to invite each family to design their dream house – what does it look like, what sort of rooms and amenities do you need, what furniture and fittings, where should it be located?'

Use and focus

The focus can be on considering realistic and unrealistic future scenarios and potential steps to get towards these. The family members mentalize each other as they consider what is important for each in terms of privacy, safe spaces, joint rooms and luxury. Questions may focus on: *'Can agreements be reached how to furnish the place? What compromises might need to be made? What do people think about the difference between dreaming your life or living your dream? Which wishes or visions have already been realized, and which are never likely to come true?'* In addition to promoting mentalizing, this activity can move families towards discussions about (realistic) hopes and dreams and how these might be achieved.

Family crest or family website

Instruction

'In the good old days, families, certainly the noble ones, had their own coat of arms which said something about their past history, their motto and their strengths. A lot of pride was invested. We would like to invite each family to design such a coat of arms for yourself. As a family think about what is special about your family, what you are proud about and what specific strengths you have. And transform all this into the coat of arms, family crest or website and if you can then think of a family motto, so much the better'.

Use and focus

The focus can be on increasing family cohesion via defining and strengthening the family's identity. Questions out to group members can include the following: *'What are each family's strengths and values? How can important past family history be contained in the coat of arms? What are the positives about each family? What might be the family motto?'* By symbolizing their strengths and values, the family has to focus their attention and negotiate. This process can reveal important family dynamics. Later similarities and differences between different coats of arms or family websites can be explored, and families invited to consider the coat of arms should look like in the future and how they might reach that point.

Family network map

Instruction

'Each family has its own structure and way of managing relationships between its members. We would like each family to map its relationships and structure. Circles and squares can represent female and male family members, respectively, and their relationships can be drawn with connecting lines. Really strong and close relationships can be drawn with double or treble lines, more distant relationships just with a dotted line. Troubled or adversarial relationships can have some flashes between them or zigzag. Remember to put in all people currently living together or even apart and anyone who is important, including grandparents, uncles and aunts. If you don't know about some of the relationships, speculate about what they might be like. If there

are any coalitions between people, invent a symbol to describe this; maybe also mark the boundaries between different generations and different branches of the family, whether you think these are rigid, flexible or too loose – and don't forget to put yourself in there as well'. Later: *'If you could only change one of the relationships on this map, which one would you go for first? How could you do that – and if it is changed, which other relationships might change automatically? And in what direction?'*

Use and focus

As this is a fairly complex task, the activity works better for families with adults and adolescents. The focus can be on significant people, interests and relationships and to show how these might complement or compete with each other. The process of making the map demands that the nature of relationships be made explicit, something that does not always happen in families. This process can lead to conversations around how people feel about different relationships and reveal new perspectives. The marking of family conflict can also support talk about previously avoided issues. Families can be encouraged to reflect on the implications of change and its effects on relationships and individuals.

Family pictures/collages

Instruction

'We would like each family to make their own picture of how you see yourselves as a family. Please put such a picture together. You can use colour pens, paint, images from magazines; you can make a collage, whatever you like'. Later: *'Now make a picture of how you would like to see your family in 6 months' time.'*

Use and focus

The process of making the picture or collage can highlight differences in family members' perspectives and key intrafamily dynamics. Questions practitioners can ask include: *'How well did they all work together when making the pictures? Who showed initiative – who didn't? Who has the main 'say'?'* The pictures or collages promote a focus on how different issues/feelings and dynamics can be expressed and recognized, sometimes making implicit mental states explicit. Families are provided with an opportunity to have their difficulties 'seen' by the rest of the group, as there can be a focus on what the picture reveals about how the family works, including their wishes, hopes and disappointments.

Family rucksack

Instruction

'Imagine that you suddenly have to leave the country you live in. You only have one rucksack for all the important family belongings, and there is only

space for five items for the whole family. Can you work out what these might be and then agree? Write down on five pieces of paper what you might wish to take – one piece of paper for each thing you want to take. Place the sheets in the rucksack.'

Use and focus

Particularly useful for families with migration histories. The focus can be on high-lighting processes of intra-familial decision making, including what is important for families and why. Questions include: *'How are decisions made? What can be left behind and what not? Who has the final say? What can one not put in a ruck-sack? Can one transport values from one culture to another? What gets lost?'* The exercise can strengthen family identity and highlight intra-family conflicts around priorities and values. Families can be asked to think about how they 'carry' their family rucksack in day-to-day life outside of the group.

Family timelines

Instruction

'We would like each family to plan their next 12 months. And the best way to do this is to have three different timelines. First, there is the timeline of the family, with all the planned and likely events, including holidays, jobs, religious festivals, exams. Then there is a second timeline: the timeline for recovery or getting rid of the prob-lems. And the third timeline is about the future if there is no change and things don't get better – what might that look like? Do this month by month.'

Use and focus

This is a suitable activity for families with children who are old enough to grasp the instruction. The activity highlights the impact of the problem on day-to-day life and mobilizes families to think about making effective changes in the near future, as it requires them to imagine a future where nothing has as yet happened. There can be a focus on the potential for change as families reflect with each other on whether their proposed recovery timeline is likely to be effective in averting the third timeline and, if not, what action they might make.

Family trees

Instruction

'We would like each family to draw their own family tree. You can use specific sym-bols to do that . . . write for each person their name, surname, age, job/work and one character trait, as well as problems or illnesses they have had. If there are any very complicated relationships between people, please mark these.'

Use and focus

Children can often become very curious to find out the story – or stories – of their family, but for parents there can be some parts of their family tree that they are not so comfortable sharing. The focus can be on examining transgenerational family patterns over time, with questions like: *'Who is similar to one another within the family? How do they feel about that? How did other family members manage a particularly problematic situation? What might grandparents and great-grandparents think about the family has grown and developed?'* Families can be encouraged to continue the talk of family stories when they get home, with a view to strengthening their identity as a family.

Note: Families with significant trauma histories may need some extra support with this activity.

Family vehicle

Instruction

'Imagine you could design an ideal vehicle to help you make your 'journey through life' – it could be a rocket, an amazing flying machine or a magic car or train or something else; there are no limits to your imagination. . . . Obviously such a means of transport needs a capable crew – like someone who cleans the vehicle, a technician, maybe a driver. You can try to draw this vehicle first if you like and then decide among yourself who has which task.'

Uses and focus

The imaginative nature of this activity can prompt families to work on 'automatic pilot' with regard to whether parents are able to actively involve their children in the activity and work together to decide the roles of family members. Later the families can be asked: *'Who is happy with the decisions and who is less so?'* Similarities and differences can be observed, and links can be made with family roles and decision making in the home.

Goal tree

Instruction

'In this activity, we would like each family to draw or paint a gigantic tree. We call it the goal tree. Each member of the family will have access to a few branches – the bigger ones are for important goals, both short-term and long-term. The smaller branches are for the smaller goals. Perhaps you should make a few large branches or even the trunk of the tree for shared family goals or goals for the parent couple. Remember to write your family name at the base of the tree and put a small basket next to it.'

Part 2: *'Now take a felt-tip pen and walk around and look at the trees. Write a compliment on a small piece of paper for each family and put it in the basket. We call these 'fertilizer buckets' because they're here to strengthen families to achieve their goals'.*

Use and focus

The focus can be on the types of goals families choose, prompting questions like: *'Are they big or small goals? Whose goals are they? How realistic are they? How can they be achieved? What help do we need to get there? What are the obstacles to these goals? What goals have already been achieved? What would have to be the first small step for the person/family to get there?'* The activity often reinforces hope and agency, and family members can be asked to identify the first step that they are going to make towards their goal before the next session.

Job references

Instruction

'Please think of one person in your family and imagine they want to apply for a job. What sort of a reference might you want to write to support the job application? Write what's positive but also what's true – otherwise they won't get the job. You can ask other people in the group to point out some of the positives if you find it difficult to think about these yourself.'

Uses and focus

There can be a focus on looking for positives and helping families to match a member's individual characteristics with the desired qualities. Helpful questions put at this point are: *'How difficult was it to find positives? How did one account for people's difficulties or problems? How does one manage praise and criticism in your family? When is praise important? Should one explicitly mention negative aspects of a person or family? What are the advantages and disadvantages of criticism?'*

Life river

Instruction

'It is possible to think about our life as a kind of river, with the springs getting together and forming a little stream which then gets bigger until it is a river. In life, as in rivers, one needs to negotiate new bends and unforeseen obstacles such as rocks and currents. Sometimes the river, our life, flows calmly, and then suddenly

we are swept along. So now imagine that this is your life as a family and you look at it from a bird's eye perspective, or imagine you sit on the riverbank and see it flowing past you. What do you see? Imagine the river has different parts, beginning from the springs, with the birth of your children – or when you met each other – and ending when it flows into the sea. If new streams flow into the river, like new additions joining the family, then mark these down. And just notice where the river, the family, flows and how it drifts'.

Use and focus

This is a particularly suitable activity for families with a trauma history. The focus can be on how riverbed changes are and were due to external influences, with questions being put to group members like: *'How can one ensure that the river remains in its riverbed in the future? How can one negotiate dangerous currents and rocks – and what might these be? Which dangerous currents have been mastered in the past and how? What challenges may lie ahead and how can they be dealt with?'* By using the metaphor, conversations about traumatic experiences can take place in a more emotionally regulated way. Previously avoided experiences can sometimes be integrated, improving autobiographical continuity and helping children make sense of their life story.

Memory lane

Instruction

'The older we get, the more we forget. Often there are memories attached to specific objects, whether it's a doll, a picture, school reports, presents from grandparents. We would like each family to bring next time no more than five personal souvenirs or relics, nothing expensive but rather something meaningful, things you value for personal reasons. And then we would like to hear something about the stories which are hidden in these objects.'

Use and focus

This is a good activity for families who 'can't remember' the past. The process of gathering the objects requires families to engage in conversations that perhaps would not otherwise be had, and the curiosity of group members can help in holding everyone's attention. The focus can be on the search for non-dominant narratives and 'unfinished business', with questions such as: *'which good stories come to mind? Is there anything hurtful? How would life be different if one had lost one object? Which objects did you think of bringing and didn't in the end? What was that about? How did you as a family agree on what to bring and what not?'* The activity promotes a focus on autobiographical continuity within the family.

Mind scanning

Instruction

'*Do you know what this is? We have drawn a diagram of a human brain. It's a kind of brain, but it has more holes than we usually have, and therefore it's also a mind. You can see that some of the holes (doctors call some of them 'ventricles') are bigger, and others are rather small. Imagine that this is your dad's head – put in there what you think his interests are, his likes and dislikes. And his fears and hopes. And I am going to give another brain to your mum: can you, Mrs F, put in there what you think goes on in your husband's head – like his thoughts and feelings – and maybe any secrets you think he has in there – maybe in the small holes. And you, Mr F, can you put in this brain diagram here what you think your wife believes goes on in your head. . . . Later we are going to have a look at what goes on in our heads. You are lucky enough to be in an ultra-modern hospital that benefits from the latest technological advances. A new piece of equipment that we have acquired produces astonishing images of the brain. It's called a brain-hyperscanner. Thanks to it, you can take an in-depth look at what's going on inside the head of a member of your family. Each of these holes is the receptacle for thoughts and emotions, and thanks to this device we can see them.*'

Variation: '*Let us imagine that this is the mind/brain of your son. Dad, can you put in the little and big holes what you think is going on there. And Mum, can you do the same on this diagram, but don't check it with your husband? And Billy, can you also fill in yet another diagram, but not what really is going on in your mind, but what you think you mum thinks are the thoughts and feelings and needs and so on?*'

Uses and focus

The mind scans can be presented to the whole group or in sub-groups and family members invited to reflect upon the accuracy of the scan. The focus can be on becoming curious about the thoughts and feelings of others, with these questions: '*How well do family members know each other? How might the scan have looked like before the illness or before problem struck the family? Which holes (ventricles) might one want to shrink or grow? How might one go about it? What would one want the mind-brain look like in 1 year's time? How might one get there?*' The activity highlights that it is not possible to ever truly 'know' what is happening in another person's brain. Yet, family members are often surprised that their brain scan is more accurate than expected.

Mood barometer

Instruction

'*We have prepared a large sheet of paper for each family, with a vertical and a horizontal line. It's to do with rating your mood and overall feelings right now and in the future. You can see that on the left, the vertical line, there is a scale from –10 to +10, and in the middle there is the 0 line. This is for each of you to fill in how you feel: –10 means really, really bad and +10 amazingly well. You probably will put your mood somewhere in between those two extremes. And then there is the horizontal (0) line – on the left of the vertical line is the past and on the right the future, and where the 0 is, that's just now. Can each family member then fill in how they feel now, with different colours so that you know who is who? And then fill in on the left when you each felt lowest in the past and put a date next to it. And when you have done it, can each of you fill in on the right of the vertical line what sort of mood you would like to be in when the work with us is finished or any other date? Once you all have done this, find another family as discussion partner and exchange ideas and experiences. And also think about one point: what would be a small step to lift the mood today – who would need to do what to make it happen?'*

Use and focus

This is a particularly suitable activity for families where affect fluctuation is prominent. The focus can be on increasing families' awareness of the different feeling states of their members and getting them to consider what changes need to be made to get to more balanced emotional states. Questions put to family members are: *'Who is/has been aware of whose moods and feelings? Who is oblivious to mood changes? Why might that be? What made it possible to lift the mood in the past?'*

Note: This activity can be done with families who have younger children, as it does not demand that they use sophisticated language around mental states. However, some additional preparation work around what is meant by feeling 'bad' and 'good' might be helpful.

Re-scripting family arguments

Instruction

'We would like you to think about a typical family argument, a situation that keeps happening over and over again and which is both annoying and a real bore to everybody. Enact this briefly and then think of a different ending for the same situation. Make it funny if you like, like a sketch in the theatre or cabaret!'

Variation: *'Write a script for the argument, and later you will choose someone from the group to act it out. You will be the director.*

Use and focus

Can be well used in work with high-conflict families. The focus can be on experimenting with different outcomes to familiar problem scenarios. When the different sketches are presented in the larger group setting afterwards, the practitioners encourage group members to comment on and suggest alternative endings or outcomes to the all-too-familiar conflicts. Families feel validated as they see the themes and even some of the specific language of their conflict reflected across the different family scripts. Being given a 'choice' about the ending in a playful way can reinforce their agency and free them from feeling 'stuck'.

Route planner

Instruction

'It's sometimes difficult to know where to start when you have a lot of problems. Here are some Post-It Notes on which each member of the family can write down a problem that they have identified and that needs to be addressed (one per Post-It Note). Then, on a large sheet of paper, divide all the problems into groups or small islands. At the end, we'll ask the parents to sit facing the sheet as if they were driving a car, with the children in the back seats. You will have to agree on the path you will take towards these islands of problems. Where do you start? Where do you go? Where do you end? Use arrows to indicate all these stages'.

Use and focus

This activity is suitable for families with adolescents and pre-adolescents. There is often curiosity initially about what each family member might write that gets the family interested in one another. The focus can be on prioritization and family cooperation, with questions such as: *'What is the best way to address problems? Should you get straight to the heart of the matter or start with a small problem? How can you involve the children in this process while keeping the decision to the parents? What happens when you want to take control of the wheel?'*

The family constitution

Instruction

'Each family has its own rules and regulations which are meant to make living together easier. It's like an unwritten constitution. Some of these rules are well known to everyone, even if nobody has ever spoken about them; others have never been mentioned and people are confused. And there is also sometimes a total absence of rules. What rules do you have in your family? Can each family list the rules that do exist or should exist, just a bit like inventing a family constitution or the 10 Family Commandments?'

Use and focus

The focus can be on making overt unspoken or non-defined rules. Families can reflect on how rules are made and discuss who reinforces them. They can be asked:

'What happens when they are broken? Is there a penal codex? Does the family think of itself as being a monarchy, dictatorship, anarchy or democracy? How do rules get adapted when children grow older or when family members leave or new ones join?' Similarities and differences can be helpful to highlight, as these often reflect different cultural value sets and can not only connect families but also expose them to alternative perspectives. The activity can also be used to strengthen family hierarchies.

Wanted posters

Instruction

'Over the next hour please make a poster/film about a theme, like feeling lonely, being frustrated or whatever else. Remember that your parents do not know your innermost feelings and thoughts. If you are able to find creative ways to represent these and the related theme, then maybe your parents and others are better able to understand you and they won't always put their foot in it. '

Uses and focus

This is a particularly helpful exercise for families containing a 'rebellious' or withdrawn young person. The focus can be on helping the young person to have the opportunity to represent their views, issues and feelings. Practitioners can field questions to the young person and parents, like: *'How can you communicate something sensitive to your parents? What did you learn about your child? How is this knowledge going to impact your relationship? Will you do anything differently? And how was it for the young people, communicating something so truthful? What would need to happen for them to do this more often at home or school?'*

C. Problem-focused activities

The activities in this section focus on specific problems and disorders that families struggle with. They aim to address the effects of 'the problem', illness or disorder on the family and larger system and aim to encourage families to experiment with viewing their difficulties differently and to develop new strategies to combat them. However, many of the activities already described above can also be tailored to address specific issues.

A matter of conscience

Instruction

'Dear families, at this stage, we think that you have acquired enough expertise to supervise us and help us find solutions for complex situations. So, here's a case

we're struggling with. It's to do with a young person; let us call him 'James'. James has just turned 18. He has been a hospital outpatient for 1½ years and is doing better: he has regained a healthy weight, he eats most meals without super-vision and he is preparing for final school exams. He's planning to study sport in the autumn, but there's no sports university in his town, so he would have to leave home. There is plenty of enthusiasm about this plan but also some anxiety that he might deteriorate if away from home. James and his parents really want to find a way forward, and they have asked us for help. Can you help? Let us start by form-ing two groups: the teenagers have to imagine what the parents are thinking about the two scenarios: James leaves home and James remains at home – what might be the fears and hopes in both scenarios. And we want the parents to imagine what the teenagers might think about both scenarios. And when you have finished this, we will ask the parents (in the role of playing teenagers) to have a discussion about the question: "Okay, if you're leaving home, how are things going to be organized?" and the teenagers (in the role of parents) "Okay, if I stay, what do you propose?"'

Use and focus

This is an activity for families containing an anorectic or psychotic teenager, and it is suitable for use towards the end of MFT. The focus can be on the issues of trust, autonomy and negotiating separation.

Adoptive meal

Instruction

'Today we want each set of parents to 'adopt' another child to see how lunch works out . . . and afterwards the children will be returned to their real parents. Please pick another child from the group. You are responsible for this child now for the next hour or so, but if you are a bit uncertain, you may ask the real parent for some advice or tips. Just ensure that the child does not sit next to their natural parent, so that all the members of the new family can get into conversation.'

Use and focus

This activity is suitable for families containing an eating-disordered young person or younger children who are 'fussy eaters'. As with the Super-nanny/super-mate activity, parents' resources and competencies to help other parents are mobilized. Parents can be asked what they have learned from the other parent that they might try at home (video feedback can help this process). The focus can be on the potential reasons (and underlying mental states) as to why one may be more successful with the child of another parent – or indeed with the parent of another child or young person. Questions that can be put to parents and children are: *'What worked with the other child and what didn't work? What worked with the other parent and what didn't work? What did you notice about your own child and their "adoptive" parents – how did they do? How do you explain the differences? How was lunch with another family for you?'*

Body image posters

Instruction

'Please draw on this wallpaper roll your own body, just as you perceive it and feel it. It should represent how you think you look. . . . When you have done so, we will ask you to lie on the paper roll and your parent will draw very tightly along the contours of your body – and then we will compare both drawings'.

Variation: *'Dear young people, we're going to ask you to create a portrait of the ideal woman for you and what you think your portrait is; you'll also do the same by imagining what these portraits are like for your mother. To do this, you'll have magazines in front of you that you can cut out, as well as felt-tip pens and sheets of paper. Mums, you do the same for yourself and your daughters.'*

Use and focus

This activity is designed for the work with anorectic teenager. The focus can be on body image distortion. Parents can be asked: *'How would it be if your brain was making you see the world in this way? How might it impact your behaviour, your relationships and complying with any treatment? How does body image distortion become driving force? Can the anorexia sufferer "correct" their distorted view of themselves? Can parents ever help with this?'*

Bully/bullied/bystander

Instruction

'We need at least four children/young persons to start this activity: one who acts as a bully, another one who is bullied and then at least two others who are bystanders. Now imagine a typical scene at break-time in school: one child gets teased by a bully, the bully escalates, other children get drawn in and watch what happens. Just enact the way you think these situations work out.'

Use and focus

This is a helpful exercise that makes sense for families with school- and peer-related issues. The focus can be on what might be going on inside the bully, the bullied person – and the thoughts and feelings of each bystander. Some of the following questions can be put to families: *'What might explain their behaviour? What are the advantages and disadvantages of intervening? Is it OK to get a teacher to help?*

How might each of them feel when they get home later that evening? Do you think they will tell anyone what happened? If no, why not? If yes, who will they tell and what do you think they would do? How can similar situations be resolved in the future?' This activity can be used to help families explore themes of aggression, shame, exclusion and fear in a more regulated way. They are under no obligation to share their own personal experiences when hypothesizing about the different characters and so find it easier to engage with social problem solving. It can also lead to discussion about whether children perceive adults – including teachers – as being protective and helpful or not.

Cost-effective dances

'As you know, these are stressful times, not only at home but also in the world at large. Just take the climate crisis and the fact that many energy sources are increasingly having to be limited, be that gas, electricity or even atomic energy. Now, the government has commissioned the famous choreographer Igor Cool to create a dance that is both energy-saving and soothing. You are going to listen to the music and the choreographer's instructions, being mindful of the current energy constraints and remember: this dance has to be energy efficient, and it has to be soothing and reduce any stress levels. And we want you to watch each other to ensure that the energy consumption of the dance remains economical'.

Use and focus

This is an activity specifically designed for families with an eating-disordered a teenager. The focus can be on: *'How is physical activity good or bad for the body and mind? How does physical activity affect our emotions? What forms of physical activity are the most effective in calming stress? What, if anything, do we gain from doing an activity together?'*

Emotion forecast

Instruction

'Most parents confronted with the same problems that you have told us about find it hard to understand, let alone predict, the states of mind of their children. Parents often feel are unprepared and helpless when yet another crisis or emotional storm happens in the family. Meteorological forecast services try to predict storms and other forms of bad and good weather so that risks of coming to harm can be reduced via being prepared and taking avoidant action. What we propose is that each parent make emotional forecasts of their child: when can you expect sunny, cloudy, rainy and stormy "weather" or times, and how do these connect with the emotions of your child? Try first to just talk to your child's other parent for 5 minutes. Then meet the parent of another child and share your thoughts for another

10 minutes, with each parent talking no longer than for about 5 minutes. When that's finished, it would be good to hear people's ideas on what works and doesn't work'.

Use and focus

This is a helpful activity for families containing children with affect regulation difficulties. The process of witnessing their parents discussing the child can help them to feel 'seen' by their parents. The shared, non-stigmatizing language about feeling states can make emotions easier to talk about. The process of parents from different families talking to each other in this structured way provides a fast learning opportunity, as they connect over similarities and compare experiences. The focus can be on sudden and fluctuating episodes of volatile affect, including anger, high levels of anxiety, depression and sensory overload. The activity can also be used to explore bi-polar presentations. Children can be asked whether they agree with their parent's extreme 'weather planning', and families can think together about how they might improve the forecast at home.

Escalation clocks

Instruction

'From time to time we all get into emotional states when everything seems to spiral out of control and when we feel that we "lose it". At those times we can become more and more angry – and it's the same with the other person(s). It's like a vicious circle, like a roundabout, and we just can't jump off. Can you each remember a time when this happened to you in the recent past? In order to work with this, we would like each person to draw the face of a big clock, with 1–12 and a line from each figure to the middle so that there are 12 segments. Let us imagine that 12 o'clock stands for it being "too late". This is when you explode or when you all start to fight. Write in that segment what happened – and then wind the clock back, hour by hour, so to speak. Work out what happened just before then (at the imaginary 11 o'clock, but this may have just been seconds before the explosion) and what happened at 10 o'clock – and so on. In this way you can trace back how things escalated – what you did or said and what someone else said and what you said or did before the other person did so – and so on. Write this all in the segments of the clock. Once you have tracked it all back, consider what you might have done differently at each point in the time tracked in order to avoid the escalation. Later you can compare your clocks with those of the other people here in the room'.

Use and focus

This is a particularly suitable activity for families where affect control is a problematic issue. The focus can be on identifying potentially escalatory interactions or situations and to consider techniques to avoid symmetrical escalations and high levels of affect dysregulation. Questions that can be put to group members include: *'What happened when you/they lost it? What did they look like to other people? Could you see it coming? At what point were you able to predict what was going to happen? How did others react? What could you have done differently at, say, 6 o'clock?'* Similarities and differences with regard to both triggers and coping mechanisms can be discussed. Strategies can be shared, and group members can be asked to look out for situations that lead to escalation between now and next time – and what they might do to prevent themselves getting to 12 o'clock.

Food collages/festive meal

Instruction

'*We are asking you to do something a bit unusual: each member of each family is asked to compose a symbolic meal, made up of cut-outs from food journals. These will be placed on plates, and we want you think about the coming Sunday lunch/ festive meal of your choice. We have plates and food magazines, and you can cut out the food that you think your child(ren) and the family should eat. Cut out all the ingredients of the food in real-size portions and stick these on the plate. So, you make your very own meal, what you would like to eat next Sunday for lunch and what the other family members should also eat'.*

Alternatively: '*Mr J, put on this plate the Sunday lunch which you think your wife would like to prepare for your daughter. And you, Mrs J, can you put on your plate the meal that you think your husband would like to prepare for your daughter? And you, Jane, can you put on your plate the meal that you think your mother would like to serve you? Next you, Mrs S: can you put on your plate the meal that you think your daughter would like you to make for her? And you, Mr S, could you put on your plate the meal that you think your daughter believes you would want your wife to make for her?'*

Use and focus

This activity works well with families containing an eating-disordered young person. A playful focus on the typically arising conflicts, anxieties and fantasies can be created, with questions such as: '*What does the young person make of all these different Sunday lunches? Which is the most and least conflict provoking meal? Who will give in first? How much would the young person need to eat for you to feel that they are putting on weight rather than losing more? If they don't eat the proposed lunch on Sunday, what is going to happen? Does the young person think their parents are over the top to expect them to eat all this? Who is right and wrong?'* Families observe familiar patterns and conflicts in other families. Observing these from a distance can allow them to take a more reflective position in relation to their own interactions, and, as a result, new perspectives can emerge. Families can finally be asked '*Having taken part in this activity will there be anything different about Sunday lunch this week?*'

Hit or smack?

Instruction

'*Many parents believe that there is nothing wrong with smacking their child occasionally if the child misbehaves. Sometimes parents are hit or kicked by their children. Often there are discussions about whether any form of physical chastisement is allowed or not. At other times people argue about the difference of a smack and a hit and whether it needs to hurt a bit or not for the child to get the message. Here is a big doll which of course can't feel any pain. We would like each of you to show how you might smack the doll if she was naughty – and also to show the difference between a smack and a hit*'.

Use and focus

This activity is helpful for families where physical chastisement is suspected. The focus can be on the impact of physical force and the search for alternative ways of managing children's challenging behaviours. Practitioners' questions can include: '*What is "too much" and what is "too little" force? What do children learn from their parents via physical punishments? What memories, good and bad, do the parents have from their own childhood? How might children's minds be affected by be hit or smacked? What do they learn?*'

Note: There are likely to be differences among parents on this topic. It can be a good opportunity for the group to both tolerate a difference in views while maintaining a boundary around not harming children. The activity can be quite emotive, especially when parents have had an experience of physical abuse as a child, when there has been previous domestic violence or when children are currently experiencing excessive chastisement.

Letter to problem/illness

Instruction

'*We would like each person to write one positive and one negative letter to "the problem". This can be a relationship difficulty, illness or disorder. When you have done so, the letters will all be put together and then distributed in such a way that each group member receives one positive and a negative letter that are not their own. These letters are then read aloud, one by one, starting with the negative ones first. A letter could start like: "Dear problem (name it), I hate you because . . . " List between five and ten reasons you hate this illness/problem. The second letter should start: "Dear problem (name it), I am grateful to you because . . . " This letter must not be sarcastic and also contain also five to ten points as the positive changes in your life which the problem/illness has brought you. Have a go now, and later we mix all the letters up, and they can be read out aloud. Let's start with the negative ones'.*

Use and focus

This is an activity for families presenting with a particular disorder or chronic problem in one or more person. Practitioners can ask: '*What are the concerns and pressures the problem produces? Which positive changes and experiences has the problem inadvertently created? What are the advantages and disadvantages of recovery? What might you – and anyone else – feel if the problem suddenly disappeared Who would miss the problem most and least?*' The focus can be on exploring ambivalence around change.

Letters from the future

Instruction

'*Think about your life at 18, 30 and 50 and imagine what may be happening in your life at that time: who you live with, your friends, what work you might be doing and where you live. Then write a letter from your future self (at these three different ages) addressing yourself at your current age. Describe your life, the course of your problem or disorder and perhaps the journey to recovery.*'

Use and focus

This is a helpful activity for families with struggling adolescents. The activity focuses on making effective changes in the near future, as it either connects them with their hopes and dreams for the future and requires that they consider what would need to change in order for them to achieve these, or it leads them to imagine a future where the long-term impact of the problem, if left unresolved, is realized. The process of sharing the hopes, dreams and fears in this indirect way can improve mentalizing and support compassion.

Links like no other

Instruction

'*Dear families, we're going to give you the chance to see the relationship between parents and children in a completely new way. After a short warm-up, we're going to use this climbing wall. First, the parents, who are linked to their child by the rope, pulley and harness, will guide their children up to the top before abseiling down. The children will then guide their parent on the wall from the ground. In the second part, parent and child will cross the wall sideways together, attached to each other by a rope'.*

Use and focus

This is an activity for families with adolescents where issues of trust are a major source of distress. The focus can be on how much one can trust each other and how competent family members are at looking after one another – and have empathy for someone who is struggling.

Note: This activity can only be used as part of a multi-family outing to an accredited climbing centre.

Press conference

Instruction

'Can we make two groups, one for children and one for the parents. If the children could come to this room and the parents stay here. Dear children, we want to ask you to help us to moderate a TV programme, called Help, My Child Has . . . (ADHD, anorexia nervosa, autism spectrum disorder etc.). You are the experts for this problem, like famous doctors and scientists or researchers . . . and you are going to talk expertly on this topic, maybe quoting from your latest books and research studies. You will each have a name displayed in front of you, such as Prof/Dr Clever . . . please answer the questions which are put to you as constructively as you can, and if you cannot answer a question, pass it on to another member of the panel'.

To the parents: 'You are all journalists and present at the TV programme, and I will be moderating the show. At the long table over there, you can see all the experts, and you, as the journalists, have the unique opportunity to ask these highly competent experts all the questions which have been preoccupying you over the years. Here, Mrs A, is the microphone; please do ask the first question . . . but the rule is not to ask the expert who is a part of your own family'.

Use and focus

This activity is popular with families containing a member suffering from a diagnosed illness or disorder. The focus can be on the symptomatic family member's lived experience and expertise. Parental curiosity is provoked as new and interesting perspectives are presented by the expert panel. The young people feel valued and taken seriously. Families can be asked: *'What are the conditions for allowing this same kind of discussion to take place at home? What have you learnt and what did you know already? How can one explain the gap between knowledge and behaviour?'*

Problem portrait

Instruction

'We would like everyone to use a sheet of this paper and think about how you would portray the problem or disorder. Let your imagination go wild – anything goes. Put your thoughts and feelings about the problem on paper'.

Use and focus

This is useful for families who over-focus or minimize a specific problem. The focus can be on the states of mind and feelings evoked by the portrait – in both the young people and adults. Making a visual representation of the problem is similar to the process of 'externalization', especially if the work of art is also given a name. This can promote a move away from locating the problem inside a person and focus on when the problem makes an appearance and how the family can work together to keep the problem in check.

Roles reversed

Instruction

'*We're going to reverse roles for a few minutes. Jenny, I suggest you come and sit at this table with Jane, your mother. Jenny, you will play the role of your mother and Jane the role of your daughter Jenny. (to Jenny) Jane, I'm sorry to tell you that your daughter is suffering from anorexia nervosa. You've come here for help, and you've been told that to help her, you have to get her to eat. And here you've got a meal in front of you that need to get your daughter to eat. (to Jane) Jenny, how old are you? You came here with your mother because you need help, but you think everything's fine. You know that your mother is going to have to feed you and that's very difficult for you. I'm going to ask the other families to watch, and we'll freeze-frame the action to try and understand what's going on in the head of this girl and her mother*'.

Variation*: 'Now I'm going to ask the anorexic person to sit down at the table with Jane and Jenny (a masked practitioner comes forward and speaks softly to the girl: 'Don't eat that, you'll get fat! She's trying to win you over, don't give in or I'll make you pay'. Then to the mother: 'Look, you're making her cry, you're a bad mother'.*

Variation: with children with ADHD or conduct disorder, same reverse role play with the following scenario: '*Kevin is in his room playing video games. His dad has to stop him and make him take a shower before he goes to bed*'.

Use and focus

This is an appropriate activity for families with a problematic child or an adolescent who is resisting parental support or guidance. There can be a focus on feeling pressured and powerless and the thoughts and feelings that are evoked.

Secret life of volcanoes

Instruction

'*Please make a colourful drawing of a volcano in a dormant state, prior to its eruption. Also draw the subterranean layers, showing what's going on underneath.*

Then make it erupt. Once you have finished the drawing, we will all talk about it and think about how to spot the volcano starting to erupt, like little rumbles and vibrations, steam coming up or the first rocks being thrown out. Imagine that you are on the volcano and you want to keep as safe as possible. What can you do? When and where can you run for shelter and stem the lava flow? When you are done, I want you to talk about the last explosion in your family. What were the warning signs?'

Use and focus

This activity can be helpful for families where members have anger issues and where physical or emotional violence tends to erupt. Questions can be put to families: *'How can you devise an "early warning system" to avoid eruptions? What role does each family member have? Is it appropriate that children should watch for signs of eruption in the adults, or is that the parents' job? Who else can be included (extended family, friends) to help understand and strengthen the early warning system?'*

Super-nanny/super-mate

Instruction

'Most of you probably will know Super-Nanny from the TV. Some people think she is very helpful; some people think she is a bit mean. Well, believe it or not, there are plenty of very helpful super-nannies here, or super-mates. And we want to give you a chance to show how good you are at helping others with their problematic children. We would like each parent to choose a partner-parent – and if you are a two-parent family, choose another two-parent family. Like Super-Nanny, you will be able to watch some problem situation that another family is struggling with, and your job is to give advice via an ear-bug to the parent who is struggling with their child. You can work out with each other what sort of input you want to have, and one of us will sit with Super-Nanny behind the one-way screen.'

Use and focus

This activity can be helpful for families containing a child with oppositional and/ or very dysregulated behaviour. The focus can be on parents' resources and competencies to help other parents. Parents are more likely to be open to support when the input comes from a peer who struggles with similar difficulties. They can be asked what they have learned that they might try at home and: *'What did you notice about the impact of any change in your behaviour on their child(ren)? What did the child notice you were doing differently?'* Parents in the helping position can experience a sense of competence, often a novel feeling.

Survival manual

Instruction

'Dear parents, after these few meetings you've spent together, you've discovered a number of tips and tricks, as well as things to avoid. We'd now like you to write a survival manual for anorexia/ADHD/ASD/schizophrenia country. Imagine what skills the poor parents who are in turmoil in this country need to have at their fingertips to help them cope. Let's start by getting into small groups of authors and dividing them up randomly: A, B, C . . . all the A's, you sit here, the B's there and so on. You are teams of very gifted authors, and you have to imagine the form and content of this survival manual. In a moment, we're going to have a meeting of the editorial committee, and we're going to have to decide what this manual is going to look like. Come on, get to work, the deadline is close'.

Use and focus

This activity can be employed in the work with families where one or more members present with a specified disorder or chronic problem: ADHD, anorexia nervosa or schizophrenia, as well as sleep disorders or communication difficulties. The manual writing can begin early on and be completed towards the end of an MFT project. Questions the practitioners can put to the manual writers include: '*What advice should be prioritized? Should we rule out a solution on principle? What would their children make of these manuals? If the children were to write a manual for parents, would it look the same or be quite different? How would your family life be different if you had read this manual 5 years ago? Which parts of the manual do you think are most important for you and your network to have to hand after the group has finished? Is the manual complete or is there more to add?'*

Survival suitcase

Instruction

'Leaving home is a time of great change in the lives of families and young people. Today we're going to ask you to imagine yourself a long time from now, on the eve of your young person's departure from home. They are leaving to study in another town; the move has already been made, you went there last weekend, and everything is ready. You took the opportunity to walk around the city as a family, which was pleasant but also a little stressful. Tonight is the last night; tomorrow your child will be gone. You decide to go and pack the suitcase with him, putting in the important things, perhaps the most symbolic ones, to help him enter his adult life. It's a special moment, the three of you alone, and it's a good time to talk honestly. We're going to ask you to build and represent the important objects together! Not the toilet paper or the toothbrush but things that you think are important to take with you into adult *life: objects that give security and strength, charged with values or emotions, so that you can grow up and become independent. Young people, you can ask your parents about the things that were important for them when they left home'.*

Use and focus

This activity can be employed when working with families with an adolescent, particularly towards the end of MFT. The focus can be on the issue of autonomy and age-appropriate relationships between young persons and their parents. Families can be asked: *'How can safety issues be addressed? What links does a young need to maintain with their family so that they can face life on their own?'*

Traps and treasures

Instruction

'We want all the child and young people to write down the advantages and disadvantages – or what's useful and counterproductive – of the illness/disorder/problem (depression, anxiety, ADHD, etc). And once you have done that, and we will place all the disadvantage papers on plastic plates, and we fold the advantage papers into tiny folds. Thank you for doing this. Now, dear families, you will be aware that sometimes the road to wellbeing is long and full of pitfalls. Here is a rope marking the start line and another marking the finish line. On the course, from the beginning to the end, there are quite a few traps, these plastic plates. You have to avoid stepping on them; otherwise you'll end up back at the starting line! And there are little treasures – the folded-over papers – to collect on the way to the finish line. The children and young people will be blindfolded and stand at the starting line. The parents will stand at the finish line and verbally guide their child to avoid the traps while collecting as many treasures as possible for their family. Afterwards, the children will guide their parents'.

Focus

This activity is for families with one or more members presenting with a specific disorder. The focus can be on exploring and naming the advantages and disadvantages of change. Families can be asked to think concretely about how they could work together to identify and keep the treasures and avoid the traps in real life – and what they might try between sessions.

Tricks the problem uses

Instruction

'Over the next hour we want to examine the 'nasty' aspects of your daughter's eating disorder by exchanging ideas and information you have all collected over the years. To fight the disorder, one needs to understand it and its power. So, let's

start and collect ideas what you have noticed about anorexia and the tricks it plays. When these difficult things happen, the question is: is this anorexia or is it your daughter speaking?'

Use and focus

A suitable activity for families with a young person suffering from anorexia nervosa, substance misuse or another defined disorder or illness. The focus is on looking at the problem as being separate from the person, how 'the problem' uses deception and manipulation and how it can be seductive.

Wigglemon

Instruction

Part 1: '*Some problems just don't give up, they stick around. Take ADD or ADHD, for example; they are both really smart. They were jealous of the Pokémon family, so they developed their own game to conquer the lives of thousands of children. The new game is called Wigglemon, and it can make children excited, restless and inattentive. Now we want each child to draw their own Wigglemon and describe the way it makes you act. When you're finished, you can show the different Wigglemons to each other'.*

Part 2: '*Now we would like the children to show their Wigglemon to their parents, and we would like each child with their parent to use a large sheet of paper to draw the Wigglemon's territory: where the Wigglemon lives, which rooms in the house he prefers, where he moves outside the house, what times and which days of the week he likes to cause trouble and so on. And when you have finished this, parents and children can then meet another family and exchange ideas and strategies like what makes the Wigglemon stronger and, more importantly, what words, emotions and behaviours can help to undermine the power of the Wigglemon.'*

Use and focus

For families with children diagnosed with ADD/ADHD, Tourette's and ODD. As with the portrait exercise, making a visual representation of the problem is similar to the process of 'externalization', and 'mapping its territory' can promote a move away from locating the problem inside a child and towards conversations about how the family can work together to keep the Wigglemon at bay. Families can be asked to reflect on what tricks they have learned together and what they might try when they get home or to school.

Stubborn donkey challenge

Instruction

'*You know that a donkey is a gentle animal when you're nice to it. But if you're rough and you force donkeys, they won't be easily led. In this activity, one by one, the children will have to guide a donkey through an obstacle course by holding it by a rope. As parents, you are not allowed to interfere with the animal but only to help your child complete the task alone'.*

Uses and focus

This an activity that suits poorly structured families. The focus can be on cooperation and managing emotions when frustration sets in. Families can be asked to mentalize the minds of donkeys (and other domestic animals) and think about what, if anything, one can learn from donkeys.

Note: This activity can only be used as part of a multi-family outing to a farm or a setting which specializes in children handling domestic animals under professional supervision.

Chapter 7

Engaging with culture
in multi-family groups

Personal and social identity

The psychotherapy literature is saturated with many descriptions and definitions of what constitutes culture and diversity, concepts that can mean something quite different to different practitioners. Multi-family work often involves individuals and families from diverse backgrounds, cultures and sub-cultures. This requires practitioners to recognize and engage with differences and inequalities, as well as to reflect on how their own cultural identity may contribute to both helpful and unhelpful dynamics in a group setting.

Several tools for identifying and reflecting on aspects of personal and social identity have been developed. These include the ADDRESSING model (Hays, 2008), which is a framework that facilitates consideration of the complexities of individual identity across the dimensions of **A**ge, developmental **D**isabilities, acquired **D**isabilities, **R**eligion, **E**thnicity, **S**exual orientation, Socioeconomic status, **I**ndigenous group membership, **N**ationality and **G**ender, and The Social GGRRAAACCEEESSS model (Burnham, 2018), which also deconstructs social identity, using the acronym as a prompt to think along different dimensions: **G**ender, **G**eography, **R**ace, **R**eligion, **A**ge, **A**bility, **A**ppearance, **C**ulture, **C**lass/Caste, **E**ducation, **E**mployment, **E**thnicity, **S**pirituality, **S**exuality and **S**exual orientation and associated interpersonal dynamics. While such tools are very helpful in that they allow examination of cultural identity, they can also raise feelings of discomfort or overwhelm on the part of the practitioner, as they highlight the complexity of cultural identity and differences related to power and privilege. It is not surprising, therefore, that despite the availability of such tools, the impact of cultural difference can get overlooked in practice. As multi-family practitioners, it is our role to understand relational patterns and to create contexts where those patterns can be changed or strengthened. Consideration of different aspects of personal and social identity is key to this process. Thus, this chapter explores some of the challenges multi-family practitioners face when it comes to engaging with culture and provides guidance with regard to navigating such challenges.

DOI: 10.4324/9781003442424-7

Challenges to engaging with culture

The term *culture* is complex and multifaceted, and it refers to shared values, norms, customs, beliefs, language and traditions that motivate individuals to identify with one another. Much of how culture organizes our thoughts, feelings and behaviours is implicit or unconscious, and, as such, it is often out of our awareness. The metaphor of an iceberg is commonly used to represent this phenomenon, with culture being analogous to an iceberg, with only about 10% of it being visible at any given time and a much larger part of it hidden beneath the surface (Hall,1976). While behaviours and practices associated with cultural identity are often observable, associated values, perceptions, attitudes and beliefs operate 'beneath the surface'. In a group that is visibly diverse, for example, where there are differences in race or age, curiosity about difference may emerge more easily and quickly. In this way a visual difference can sometimes act as a prompt or a 'way in' to culture. However, there are several dimensions of culture, for example, sexual or gender identity, that may not be evident.

Practice example:

In a multi-family group involving carers and young babies, group members' different social and cultural identities may mean that there are different beliefs, both amongst the parents and practitioners, about the position a baby or child should occupy within a family and the amount of focus or attention they should be given by their carers. These beliefs are likely to have a significant impact both at an intra- and inter-personal level. However, unless MFT practitioners are able to make such differences explicit, the resulting impact on group process will remain unaddressed.

Thus, it can be hard for practitioners to *see* the impact of cultural identity on both inter- and intra-personal communication in a group. In the absence of visual prompts, the first challenge is to create contexts that allow relevant dimensions of identity to become 'visible': Culture has to be 'seen' before it can be explored.

A second challenge is associated with the fact that culture is in a dynamic and constant state of flux over time, place and person. It is a broad concept with many interrelated dimensions that shift and change their influence across different contexts. Different aspects of personal and social identity within the same person become more or less relevant in different settings. Related to this is the idea of 'intersectionality', that is, understanding how a person's various social and political identities co-exist to both organize behaviour and create different modes of discrimination and privilege. Thus, a second challenge faced by MFT practitioners is the need to temporarily hold culture 'still' in order to focus on a particular aspect of identity.

Practice example

A group discussion or MFT activity about the social expectations of male and female carers in the UK is likely to look different now to how it would have looked 50 years ago or how it might currently look in some Middle Eastern or Southeast Asian countries. Gender may be the 'highest context marker' (Cronen et al., 1979) for a man discussing the roles of fathers in a group with other parents from different religious backgrounds. However, his Muslim faith may exert a stronger organizing function when he is communicating about the same issue amongst a group of Muslim parents. Same-sex parents may feel inhibited to share their views about gender roles during a multifamily group discussion about the social expectations of male and female carers if this discussion is heteronormative.

A third challenge faced by practitioners is the need to balance the benefits of engaging with cultural difference with the risk this may pose to group cohesion or therapeutic focus. Practitioners actively look for commonalities between families, with the aim of reducing shame and stigma and freeing them up to mobilize their own and each other's ideas and strengths. At the same time, they strive to create contexts where different perspectives can be experienced in a way that is 'acceptable' to group members and without undermining the unity of the group or inadvertently reinforcing divisions. The fourth challenge for the practitioner is to assess the potential risks and benefits of engaging with culture in the moment and to judge whether it is helpful to bring cultural differences to the group context or to follow this up with families at a later stage either individually or in sub-groups. Factors such as the phase of the group's life and the nature of the differences are relevant when making such decisions.

Practice example

An activity commonly used in multi-family groups is the 'cross-fostering' exercise (see Chapter 3). Here parents take care of another family's child for a short period of time, usually with a focus on a particular task. This activity is sometimes embraced more readily by parents from cultural backgrounds where a communal approach to childcare is adopted than with those who have been brought up with an individual-focused family unit approach to childcare. A practitioner may observe differences in engagement across the group as a result of such cultural difference(s). However, the advantages of explicitly exploring such differences will need to be balanced with the disadvantages. Taking up the difference may 'level out' group engagement and could lead to families being helpfully exposed to diverse views and experiences. However, diverting the focus from the original activity may result in reduced gains for those families who engaged more readily.

Finally, and possibly most challenging, is the fact that engagement with culture and diversity can require the practitioners to address discriminatory behaviours 'head on'. While MFT can offer an opportunity to tackle prejudice by bringing people from different cultures together and providing lived experience that may challenge existing views, this very same context can also trigger prejudiced behaviour. Explicit examples of this – such as a group member using a derogatory term about aspects of culture towards another group member – are in some ways easier to address than behaviour that reflects a subtle or implicit undercurrent of prejudice. Where discrimination is explicit, it can be noticed, named and responded to. The more cohesive a multifamily group becomes, the more likely it is it that group members will themselves respond to prejudices and challenge related behaviours or comments. Groundwork such as the group establishing rules around respect for one another facilitates such support. If a prejudicial comment is made by a child, it is the role of the practitioners to create a context where the child's parents can respond. This may also involve other group members. However, if they are not actively challenging discriminatory behaviour, practitioners need to intervene in order to maintain a sense of safety and holding. Often practitioners' own ability to mentalize can be thrown offline in such instances. When this is the case, they may need to buy themselves some time to self-regulate and think about how to respond most helpfully. Both the initiator(s) and the target(s) of the communication need to be responded to in a way that minimizes shame and promotes mentalizing.

Prejudicial behaviours can often be subtle or implicit, and they are sometimes referred to as 'microaggressions'. There are two main reasons practitioners may find it difficult to take up issues at this level in the moment. First, the discriminatory behaviour may not be noticed by the practitioners because it is very subtle, because it aligns with their own subconscious biases or because the practitioners' privilege may make it hard for them to recognize the impact of the behaviour. Second, the practitioners may notice the behaviour but feel too anxious to address it, maybe because they don't want to risk de-stabilizing the group, they want to avoid causing offence, it is connected with their own discomfort or because they themselves feel oppressed by the dominant discourse. While there are many strong reasons prejudice, however subtle, may go unnoticed or unchallenged in a group setting, these do not serve to justify avoiding the issue. If practitioners do *not* engage with these dynamics, they are, implicitly, affirming them. It is important to acknowledge that practitioners themselves can also, unintentionally, perpetrate bias and microaggressions (Owen et al., 2014). Thus, the challenge for practitioners is to develop both an awareness and willingness to actively take up prejudiced behaviour that may be missed or minimized as a result of their own cultural identity and associated biases, vulnerabilities and discomfort.

Practice examples:

A British, atheist father makes an Islamophobic comment about terrorist attacks directed at a Pakistani father in the group.

A professional middle-class mother behaves in a condescending manner towards a younger and less educated parent, 'explaining' something about how it is important for children to have a balanced diet.

A white parent comments to the rest of the group 'Look at his hair! Isn't it amazing!' about the afro-textured hair of a Black child in a way that leaves him and his mother feeling othered.

Box 6 summarizes the challenges practitioners can meet in their work with multifamily groups, and it provides suggestions for how to address these.

Box 6   Challenges to engaging with culture in MF groups

Challenge	Context needed to engage the group
Many dimensions of culture and associated values and beliefs are not visible	Practitioner identifies relevant dimensions of culture which are not visible and makes them explicit so that they can be explored
Culture is dynamic and multifaceted	Practitioner focuses attention on one specific dimension of culture and/or actively explores the relationship between different components of identity
Focusing on cultural difference can have a destabilizing effect in the moment	Practitioner balances the benefits of engaging in the moment (as opposed to at a later stage) with the risks associated with amplifying divisions or moving away from a problem focus
Practitioner's identity, associated biases or discomfort prevent(s) engagement with prejudice behaviour	Practitioner can reflect on their own identity and responses to the group and its members, adopting a culturally humble position

Cultural humility as a foundation for engagement

The ability to reflect on one's own cultural identity and associated responses to the group and group members is necessary to address all the challenges to engagement identified previously. Such engagement is relational and recursive. It requires an acceptance that group members and practitioners each hold their own conscious and unconscious values, biases and stereotypes. These are taught through lived experiences and have a strong influence over each person's thoughts, feelings and behaviours at any given moment. To strictly engage with culture in MF groups, it is not enough to look at the interaction between group members; one also must understand the lens through which one is seeing and responding to it. One way of developing self-reflexive practice is via the multi-cultural orientation framework (MCO; Owen et al., 2011, Davis et al., 2018). It focuses on therapeutic process and how the cultural worldviews, values and beliefs of families and practitioners interact and influence one another. The framework identifies an orienting attitude, *cultural humility*, a concept developed more than 25 years ago (Tervalon & Murray-Garcia, 1998). It describes the process of entering a relationship with the intention of honouring the others' beliefs, customs and values and involves *intrapersonal humility* (having a more or less accurate view of oneself – particularly about one's limitations) and *interpersonally humility* (being other-oriented rather than self-centred, marked especially by a lack of feeling superior). It entails an ongoing process of self-exploration and self-critique, combined with a willingness to learn from others. Owen et al. (2011) explain how, unlike the concept of *cultural competence*, cultural humility de-emphasizes cultural knowledge and competency and places greater emphasis on:

- the long-term cultivation of self-understanding and self-critique
- an awareness of one's own implicit biases
- the promotion of interpersonal sensitivity and openness to learning
- the appreciation of intracultural variation and individuality

Being culturally humble involves an acceptance that families belonging to different cultural groups may perceive or directly experience misalignment between their views and priorities and those of the practitioners (including beliefs about pathology and health), which may, in turn, impact engagement. It also involves an acceptance that practitioners cannot be 'neutral'. Therapy is a culturally laden process, and practitioners are likely to experience incongruences between their personal values and those of some group members. Culturally humble practitioners recognize that they are usually in a position of power relative to the families and thus have greater control over the direction of the work. Finally, to be culturally humble, practitioners need to recognize that families often enter the work by being vigilant and worried about their ability to trust due to adverse past experiences and perceived differences in values and beliefs (Stubbe, 2020). The MCO framework describes how one can express cultural humility by recognizing and engaging with *cultural opportunities* and *cultural comfort.*

Cultural opportunities and cultural comfort

In any MF group, opportunities which allow exploration of cultural identity will arise continuously. These occur when group members talk about their experience, beliefs or values in ways that provide opportunities to explore their culture in more depth. Alternatively, practitioners can initiate cultural opportunities via conversations or activities when they feel these are warranted, though it is important that they do so naturally and in an attuned way and that they do not feel forced or inauthentic. Both responding to and initiating cultural opportunities requires a stance of cultural comfort – the practitioner's ability to self-regulate while engaging with culture. To be comfortable, practitioners need some understanding of their own thoughts, feelings and behaviours in relation to any specific content. They should be able to recognize and respond when feelings of discomfort arise within them and actively seek feedback from their co-therapist and members of the group in response to any interventions made. Space for practitioners to explore and understand their own cultural identity, biases and potential areas of cultural discomfort, as well as a general interest in culture, are required to develop a sense of cultural confidence. All this is a lifelong, ongoing, continuous process, supported by training, supervision, team working and personal exploration. Tools such as the Social GGR-RAAACCEEESSS model (Burnham, 2018) and the ADDRESSING model (Hays, 2008) described earlier in this chapter can provide a useful starting point. More comprehensive practice guidelines, such as Asnaani's seven applied guidelines for evidence-based practice (Asnaani, 2023), can be adopted by practitioners and teams who want to integrate a stance of cultural humility across their practice (see Box 7).

Box 7   Guidelines to support culturally humble practice
(Asnaani, 2023)

1. Exploring your own cultural identity, beliefs and biases before providing therapy
2. Practicing cultural humility as a continuous process
3. Balancing culturally informed and individualized assessment of the presenting problem
4. Engaging in self-education about specific cultural norms using a variety of sources
5. Addressing stigma and other cultural barriers to psychological treatment
6. Exploring the impact of discrimination and microaggressions on therapy
7. Identifying and incorporating cultural strengths and resources into treatment

---

Co-work helps to facilitates cultural humility, in that the practitioner in the observer role can support the active practitioner to spot cultural opportunities and to identify when cultural discomfort may have led them avoid an issue or to respond in an unhelpful way. When this happens, the active practitioner can adopt a position of cultural humility by marking the fact that they may have missed something important and returning to it either immediately or at a later point.

Practice example: Cultural humility

A practitioner and her co-worker are using the MCO model to consider the potential impact of differences in formal education amongst parents of a multi-family school group. They have met all the families, but the group has not yet started. They note how the parents who are formally educated also tend to be more verbal and wealthier than the less educated parents. The practitioners think more generally about issues to do with social class and the power imbalance between younger, less educated group members and more mature, middle-class members (including themselves). They recognize that their beliefs about a 'good outcome' are influenced by their life experiences and their professional training and may be more closely aligned with the formally educated parents. They also recognize the potential for missing opportunities to engage with issues of social class because these are not familiar to them or because they may experience guilt (and therefore cultural discomfort) associated with their own privilege. As a result of these reflections, the practitioners pay particular attention to issues of trust with the younger, less educated group during the assessment and the initial stages of the group. They make it explicit to the whole group that people can have different motivations and aims for attending MFT and ensure that they are proactive in listening for views that are different to theirs. They are curious about differences associated with social class. During a check-in, one of the more formally educated parents begins talking about changes she has noticed in her interaction with her child, namely that he is listening more to her at home. She thinks this is because she is spending more quality time with him. She reads a book to him each night, and on the way home from school they stop off for a hot chocolate. She is taking time to listen to him when things go wrong rather than 'jumping in'. The active practitioner is happy to hear about the progress, asking questions and hoping that other parents will be able to benefit from this exchange. The mother's account takes quite a lot of the space. One of the younger mothers is quiet and offers little when it comes to her turn. The active practitioner does not want to pressure this mother, who looks tired, and is keen to introduce the MF activity she and her colleague have planned. However, the observing practitioner takes this moment to notice the younger mother's lack of engagement, reflecting: 'Maybe this is because she doesn't have much to say, or could it be something else? A bad week?' The active practitioner comes back to her and makes a comment about the group being there to support each other through good and bad weeks. The mother shrugs. The practitioner asks if any of the other parents know something about how it has been for her this week? Another of the younger parents remarks that she thinks she has had a tough week. The practitioner invites her again to share and apologizes for not picking up on this first time round. The mother begins talking about her work in some detail. The practitioner initially finds it hard to see the relevance of her account, but 'leans in' to the conversation, listening and asking some curious questions. It is not long before it becomes apparent that the stress and pressure that the parent is experiencing at work, due to long hours and difficult conditions, mean that she has found it particularly difficult to manage her son's behaviour. Because of her personal circumstances it is not possible for her to change jobs or give up work, so she feels quite hopeless about things getting better. Other group members can relate to aspects of her experience, and she feels validated. The practitioners resists the temptation to get into 'problem solving' mode because of the discomfort they feel associated with her own privilege and stay with the stress and injustice of the situation. The middle-class mother who spoke earlier of her success comes alongside the younger parent, putting her arm around her, and admires her strength and commitment to her son under such difficult conditions, stating that she would not be able to manage half as well in the same situation.

Bringing culture into the room: MFT activities to promote engagement

In MFT groups it often becomes apparent that an aspect of culture is particularly relevant because it has an impact on group cohesion (positive or negative), it is of therapeutic relevance or for both reasons. At these points practitioners may choose to create a cultural opportunity by introducing a specific activity. Well-timed and pitched MFT activities which reflect a position of cultural humility can provide an opportunity to address many of the challenges identified in Box 6. They enable the practitioners to make specific dimensions of culture 'visible' and to hold the group's focus still for a short moment in time to allow exploration of specific dimension(s). The opportunity for careful planning and considering the potential pros and cons of introducing the activity on group stability increases its chances of success. Finally, the structure and timing of the exercise and the adoption of a playful stance are emotionally regulating components of the intervention and thus maximize the chance that the chosen activity will be helpful. When introducing an activity that may risk destabilizing the group, it can help to remind families of the rules that they made when the group first started, for example, respecting one another. They can then be asked how they could ensure that these rules are upheld during an activity that might raise strong feelings or controversial views. This signals that group members (also) have a role and responsibility for sustaining a safe work context. At the same time, the practitioners have to be prepared to intervene, if necessary, to maintain a safe space for the whole group.

Practice example: Geography sculpt

Two UK-based practitioners who are running a MFT group for families in care proceeding have noticed themes of identity and belonging becoming pertinent. So far, they have not directly engaged with the theme, as they have found it hard to 'get hold' of it in the moment. However, they have 'bookmarked' their observations and feel that the group is at a stage where it is robust enough for them to explore it directly via a multi-family activity. The next week they introduce the geography sculpt. They begin by orienting the group to the agreement they made with each other at the outset to be respectful to one another and ask the families to make a big space in the room by putting all the chairs to the side. When the room is clear, the active therapist stands in the middle and explains that the room is a map of the world and that they are standing in their current location (e.g., London, Paris, Berlin, New York) and points in the direction of north, south, east and west. They explain that they would like everyone in the room to stand in the place where they were born. They only have 5 minutes to do this. The families move around asking one another 'where' they are and positioning themselves accordingly. There are a lot of adjustments. A parent from Australia squeezes herself against the far wall, and two other parents work together to 'find' Bangladesh. Some parents from the same family stand in different places. Most of the children were born in London and so stay in the middle, but some of them go and stand with their parents in their country of origin. After 5 minutes the practitioner asks the group to stay where it is, explaining that it doesn't matter if it is not completely accurate, and asks them to look around the room as a way to focus attention from self to other and promote curiosity. They then approach a well-engaged 10-year-old boy who is standing with his parents to the right of the room. With a fake microphone in their hand, the practitioner puts on the voice of a television presenter and explains they are making a TV programme 'for the BBC'. They say, 'May I ask you, where is it that you are standing right now?', passing the microphone to the boy. The boy replies that he is in Ghana. The practitioner takes back the microphone, saying, 'May I ask, how long did you live in Ghana for?' The boy replies until he was 5, and the practitioner asks him what the weather is like there. He says mostly very hot, looking to his parents for confirmation, which they give him. The practitioner then hands the microphone to the boy, explaining that it is his turn to be the TV presenter. 'Look around the room. Who would you like to interview, and what would you like to ask them?' The boy takes the microphone and is quickly drawn to the Australian parent who is squashed against the wall, asking her where she is and what it is like there. After his brief interview, the practitioner prompts him to pass the microphone to the Australian parent, and it is her turn to be the presenter. After a few 'interviews' of this kind, group members are asked to position themselves again in response to a different instruction: 'Please place yourself where your grandparents were born' (children may need help from their parents with this). Again, after the families have positioned themselves, group members can interview each other. Finally, families can be asked where they would like to be living in 20 years and again interview one another about their positions: where will they be living? Why? What will need to happen between now and then to make this dream come true? The practitioner is careful to keep the energy going, staying within the time frame and ensuring engagement across the group by asking 'presenters' to approach someone who has not yet been interviewed. This activity can bring forth stories of culture, migration and difference and can stimulate curiosity, narrative building and group integration.

Another helpful activity commonly used to engage with dimensions of cultural identity is the Family Crest. Here families are remined that, a long time ago, noble families in some countries would have a 'coat of arms', represented by a crest, which said something about their history, their 'motto' and their strengths. Families are invited to design a family crest for themselves, to think about what is special about their family, what values are important to them (to make a 'motto') and what strengths they have. When the time is up, they are invited to display their family crest to the rest of the group, who can ask questions. This activity can facilitate the exploration of family values in a safe and positive way. Similarities and differences can be noticed and curiosity evoked.

A more focused activity that can be used to engage with specific dimensions of culture is the 'ribbon game'. Here the practitioners use ribbons as a way of 'externalizing' a dimension of culture. For example, if the dimension to be explored was faith, the practitioners would ask the group members to stand in a circle and pass round a ball of ribbon and request them to connect themselves to the ribbon in ways that show their relationship with faith. The practitioners explain: '*If I held faith in my heart and it was very important to me, I might wrap it round my chest like this, maybe multiple times. . . . If I didn't have a faith, and only learnt about it at school and heard about it in the news, I might wrap it round my head like this. . . . If I felt my faith linked me with my family, I might put it round my hand like this. . . . If I didn't feel any connection with faith, I might not touch the ribbon at all . . .*' and so on. If there are families where engagement with faith is a particular issue or groups where cohesion is not strong enough to manage this activity as a whole, each family can be given their own ribbon to complete the same task. At the end of the activity, the group members look around and explore with each other how they have connected themselves to the ribbons and why. Again, similarities and differences can be seen and investigated. Photos can be taken if it is difficult for families to hold their position with the ribbon or if it is felt that there would be more self-regulation and therefore better reflection if one were to look at photos rather than the 'live' representation in the room. This activity can be employed in many ways, with the ribbons symbolizing diverse aspects of culture. For example, differently coloured ribbons can be used at the same time to represent multiple dimensions of culture. As this is quite an abstract activity, parents often need to help younger children to understand it, which usually involves them having to find out what their children already know about faith, leading frequently to conversations they may have never had before.

Bringing culture into the room: Working in the moment

While well-pitched multi-family activities can be a productive and relatively safe means to engage with culture, 'bookmarking' and returning to particular themes is not always possible or even appropriate, particularly when unconscious bias or plain prejudice is at play. In these situations, practitioners will need to respond in the moment by blocking and addressing the concerning communications or behaviours, seeking the assistance of group members. If the practitioners miss this opportunity or feel unable to directly challenge bias in a potentially helpful way, they can decide to try and create a context which counters the perceived power imbalance. This involves addressing all four domains of context making (see Chapter 3): a) *the person context* (for example, by privileging the voice or position of the marginalized group member and separating parents and children in parallel groups so that more adult conversations can be had), b) *the activity context* (for example, by engaging the group in an activity that in some way challenges discrimination or by creating a focus on the specific dimension of culture so that it can be opened up more broadly for the group), c) *the place context* (for example, by working with individual families in different rooms so that private conversations can be had between them); and d) *the time context* (for example, by shutting down a conversation and moving the group on to an activity with the intention of coming back to the issue in some way later on in the group). Decisions about which specific context to make are dependent on the needs of the group. Sometimes, in such situations, it can be hard to 'think on your feet', and here the practitioners might try to find a few minutes aside from the families to think together. However, if the practitioners decide to proceed, it is usually advisable to find 1:1 time with the marginalized group member(s) to let them know what they noticed, to check whether their experience of the seemingly problematic situation matched and to ascertain the group member's views on how it should be responded to. Sometimes such conversations involve whole families and sometimes just adults. A conversation may also need to take place with the group member who behaved in a discriminatory way, depending on the situation and the relative success of the practitioners' attempts to address the behaviour in the moment. This conversation would aim to help the group member to mentalize the impact of their communication and/or behaviour while being sensitive to the person's feelings of shame that may be evoked. This can be done, for example, by recognizing that any negative impact may have been unintentional. Discriminatory communications or behaviours displayed by children are best managed if their parents are supported either by the whole group, by one or two other families or the practitioner alone. The focus is on helping their children to become aware of the impact of discrimination and understand the thoughts and feelings of the affected person(s).

Practice example: Context making to address marginalization

Practitioners providing a multi-family group to support adoptive parents with a traumatized child in Denmark observe a sub-group of families that dominate the conversation about what constitutes 'good parenting'. Almost all families are white; they were born in Denmark and have strongly held views about the subject. In the group there is also one refugee family from Afghanistan and one family with same-sex parents (two mothers) who are not contributing to the discussion. Despite the practitioners' repeated attempts to bring the marginalized group members into the conversation, they remain silent. The practitioners then decide to try to create equal space for different narratives by engaging the group in an activity with parents being asked to take time to think about parenting practices from their own history and culture and to identify three which they intend to continue as well as three which they wish to discontinue – and to write these on two Post-It Notes. The parents are then each given space to share what they have written on the Post-It Notes with the rest of the group. If they wish, they can throw the practices that they wish to discard into a bin prominently displayed in the middle of the room or discard them at the end of the meeting. By occupying a position of cultural humility and allowing equal time and value in relation to each parent's stories, this activity challenges marginalization and stimulates curiosity about similarities and differences across the group.

MFT and social justice

There is much talk amongst mental health providers about the importance of ensuring equity of care regarding different cultural and social groups. However, with much evidence indicating that inequality is significant and that little progress has been made in diminishing this gap (Bansal et al., 2022; Campion et al., 2013), it could be argued that a more socially active position is required. With its focus on context and its roots in reflexive practice, MFT provides a model that enables practitioners to work proactively with a view to recognizing inequalities from the outset and creating a more socially just provision. Practitioners are open to alternative ways of constructing mental health and recovery and pay careful attention to how different dimensions of identity can influence health, coping strategies, barriers and facilitators to engagement. This way they can empower families to bring all parts of themselves to a group and become 'equal partners in their own recovery' (Asnaani, 2023). This principle, of empowering families to engage in their own recovery, is at the heart of MFT and, as such, is as important as any specific technique or activity described in this book.

Chapter 8

MFT projects in mental health settings

Over the past 50 years, many different MFT projects have been developed, with innovative ones emerging as we write. To describe the many different applications of MFT in diverse mental health settings is beyond the scope of this book, and in this chapter, we present only a few examples of projects, hopefully serving as useful illustrations of what MFT for specific presentations might consist of. Details of the exercises we refer to can be found in Chapter 6. Of course, there are plenty of different ways of delivering MFT for any defined problem or disorder, and these will be determined by a team's orientation and creativity, as well as by contextual issues such as resources, location, finance, institutional dynamics and more. MFT projects can be very structured and do exist in tightly manualized versions, thereby providing a framework with a predetermined sequence of interventions. Yet other projects are more loosely organized, with both content and process of each session being co-constructed with group members and being reviewed and perhaps newly invented from session to session.

In the diverse services involved in managing mental health issues, be that psychiatry, psychology or psychotherapy, diagnoses play a major role, and in this chapter, we describe several disorder-focused MFT projects. Different from these are generic MFT projects involving, for example, all young persons admitted to a psychiatric in-patient hospital unit, irrespective of their diagnoses. The common denominator for these families is the fact that one of their children is an in-patient and is temporarily excluded from ordinary family life, with resulting dynamics that can benefit from mutual exploration. Here MFT work takes place mid-week each week, for about 90 minutes, with all the current in-patients having their families arrive in the afternoon and taking part in a multi-family event. This is obviously an open group with its participants coming and going as new admissions arrive and other patients get discharged. The focus of these groups is often on how to improve the ward living environment, how to give patients more of a voice, how to involve their primary carers more in medical and social decision making and how to manage being away from one's family and then being reintegrated.

There is another generic application of MFT in mental health services: it is the result of the current state of child and adolescent mental health services, with its increasingly long waiting lists. Several clinical teams in different parts of Europe

DOI: 10.4324/9781003442424-8

have developed MFT projects to deal with waiting lists. These are open groups, taking place on a fortnightly basis and each lasting between 90 and 120 minutes, bringing together families either with children aged 5 to 11 or families with adolescents age 12 to 17. MFT groups usually are divided into those with children presenting with neurodevelopmental disorders, conduct disorders, emotional disorders or eating disorders. Practitioners get families to share problems, to talk about attempted solutions, to advise each other about successful strategies and to share their anxieties.

1. Taming ADHD

Overview and format

The term 'neurodiversity' was first introduced in the 1990s to fight stigma associated with attention deficit hyperactivity disorder (ADHD), autistic spectrum disorder (ASD), dyslexia and other 'neurodevelopmental disorders'. It describes the different ways people's brains may work and implies that there are no 'normal' or 'correct' ways in which this happens but that there is a range of modes how people perceive and respond to others and the world at large. It is acknowledged that persons with neurodiverse conditions, like autism/autistic spectrum disorder, may find it difficult to do some of the things they want to do and achieve given that the world is organized around neurotypical people, and this has resulted in various interventions which have been developed to reduce the difficulties and symptomologies. Embracing and encouraging these differences is important, as well as focusing on a person's talents and strengths. Diverse situations and environments can contribute to the difficulties of neurodiverse people, like school classrooms or specific social activities (e.g., children's birthday parties) where they feel misunderstood and excluded. 'Neurodiversity' can also become part of an identity, particularly in teenagers who are struggling socially; this identity can create valuable shared connections to others who equally identify as being neurodiverse and who also experience, think and process 'outside the box'. MFT is an obvious intervention bringing together families containing one or more neurodiverse members (Ma et al., 2017, 2018). The following is an example of a possible MFT project to address families with a child with diagnosed or suspected attention deficit hyperactivity disorder or attention deficit disorder (ADD).

The 8-week 'Taming ADHD' programme is suitable for families with children aged 5 to 11 years. Children attend each session with at least one of their primary carers and siblings (if of similar ages). Sessions are conducted by two MFT practitioners. Most sessions start with an *ice-breaker* activity and/or *speed dating*, with the children sitting in the inside circle and the parents in the outside circle. Specific themes are introduced via viewing video examples, followed by reflective discussions, mini role-plays and experimentation. Homework tasks are provided so that families can continue the work between MFT sessions.

Session 1: Contextualizing ADHD symptomatology

Collaborative psychoeducation: what is ADHD/ADD? What are the strengths, symptoms, causes and remedies? What do group members already know about it? This is done in small discussion groups, involving parents in parallel with children. Each group is invited to feed back the main points, and then two children and two parents are invited to summarize what has been said and to prepare a mini-lecture on the subject. One lecture is then given by a child 'professor', the other by a parent 'professor'. Each family is then asked to provide a map of when and where which symptoms happen. The results are presented to the larger group, and members are invited to speculate how and why the symptoms fluctuate. They are also asked to define what is 'normal' and what is 'pathological' hyperactivity – and how 'it' can be predicted, managed and prevented/channelled. A homework task is set: the families are asked to search for more information on ADHD and related disorders via the Internet, magazines and books and also to find out information from friends.

Session 2: Naming and re-naming problematic behaviours

Video examples of seeming ADHD 'symptomatic' behaviours are shown. Parents and children, together or in parallel groups, label (with adjectives) what they see and then speculate about the respective causations of the observed behaviours. Group members are encouraged to consider what 'angry', 'bored', 'fidgety', 'disruptive', 'oppositional' behaviours would look (and sound) like. Children are requested to enact these, and the observing parents are asked how they differentiate between 'real' ADHD behaviours and other forms problematic behaviours (e.g., attention-seeking, angry or oppositional behaviours). This is followed by a playful MFT activity that focuses on 'control' and 'self-control' issues (e.g., 'mindless robot', *'remote control'*, 'magic self-control buttons'). Towards the end of the group participants are asked, in small groups, to draw up guidelines about how to diagnose and treat 'real' and 'fake' ADHD presentations. Homework: Identify two situations which were definitely 'real ADHD' and two situations which were definitely 'fake ADHD' and report back next session.

Session 3: Externalizing ADHD

The aim for this session is to diminish the relative influence of problematic behaviours linked with ADHD/ADD on the child. This is done via externalization techniques (see Chapter 3), separating the problematic ADHD behaviour from the child, with a message given along the lines of: *'we like you, but we don't like this behaviour'*. Each family has the task to personify problematic ADHD behaviour and give it an appropriate name, such as 'Mr Temper', 'Bob', 'red mist', and to develop a character for it. Families present their ideas to each other and develop group strategies to combat 'Bob' – who can also be physically represented by a doll or another object. Families can then role play reducing Bob's power, make fun of him and celebrate success with a little party. The activity *Wigglemon* can also be employed. Homework for families: consider defeating Bob on uneven days of the week.

Session 4: Putting feelings on the map

Searching for, and naming, different feeling states. This can be done by 'live' emotion snapshots and the subsequent guessing of feeling states, as well as by activities such as Frozen *Frozen problems*, *Body Feelings* and *Photo Stories*. Parents should participate, too. The exploration of cross-cultural displays of feeling states and their accompanying narratives can be further undertaken.

Session 5: Regulating affect

Viewing of video examples of person(s) in high arousal and group discussion on its effects on children, parents and significant others. Increased physical arousal can then be created in the children by, for example, involving them in circuit training, bean bag throwing or balloon bursting, followed by a competition as to which child is best and/or fastest at down-regulating their states, as measured by their ability to engage immediately in an activity that requires full concentration (e.g., math tasks, *Wrong-hand writing* activity).

Session 6: Addressing hypothetical scenarios

The strengths and difficulties associated with ADHD are revisited. The strengths are celebrated and the difficulties identified as a focus for change. A range of settings are identified in which symptomatic/problematic behaviours and interactions are likely to occur, such as in the classroom, at break time, during a school trip, when parental friends are visiting the family home. Typical scenarios are presented and then enacted via mini-role plays. Observations, suggestions and strategies are invited and then implemented during the next phase of the role play. Group members are encouraged to devise a 'Taming ADHD Manual' or 'ADHD First Aid Box', describing how to deal with such or similar scenarios.

Session 7: Changing family life style

A collaborative psychoeducation session, with parents exchanging experiences and thoughts about diets, balanced food, elimination of toxins, adding supplements and so on. They can be encouraged to use the Internet to stimulate ideas. They are also invited to consider the virtues of 'fresh air' and regular physical exercise. The focus can be on improving the learning environment at home, as well as considering imposing restrictions on social media use, implementing regular bedtimes and other routines. Homework: each family to provide a design of 'optimal family health'.

Session 8: Relapse prevention

The last session focuses on spotting potential deterioration of behaviours, that is, 'lapses' and 'relapses', and identifying warning signs as well as considering how to respond. This can be done by exploring different hypothetical scenarios. The focus is then shifted to situations where ADHD provides strength and how to build more opportunities where it can become a 'friend'. During the last part of this final session, the 'Taming ADHD' manual can be revisited and completed, including how to manage both the positive and negative aspects of the diagnosis.

2. Living with autism

Overview and format

Different MFT programmes for working with families containing an autistic child have been developed both for children with high-functioning autistic spectrum disorder (previously known as 'Asperger's syndrome') as well as for children with severe or profound autism (level 3 'classic autism', as originally described by Kanner, 1943). MFT work with children containing a child with high-functioning autism tends to be quite similar to the MFT work with ADHD, as described, with the obvious difference that the identified problem is 'high-functioning ASD'. An eight-session format has shown to be helpful for these families, though components of the following programme can also be adapted and incorporated as needed.

'Living with Autism' takes place in fortnightly intervals, with each session lasting 2 hours (see also Nashef & Mohr, 2017). It is designed for families with a child presenting with profound early autism, being nonverbal or minimally verbal and presenting with significant cognitive deficits, with an IQ of less than 50. The children need intensive help for managing all daily living tasks, from having their meals prepared and being fed to being washed and dressed and requiring round-the-clock support and supervision to be safe. 'Living with Autism' can be applied for two separate age groups: children aged 2 to 5 years and children aged 6 to 9 years. The children attend each session with at least one parent or main carer. Two sessions are also attended by siblings and other members of the wider family support network. Two rooms are needed to allow for parallel parents' and children's groups to take place. A minimum of three MFT practitioners is required: one (or two) for the parents' group and two for the children's group. Familiar objects and toys are needed, in addition to illuminated toys, magnifying glasses and binoculars and visual supports (pictograms, TEACCH).

The *first hour* consists of a parallel parents' and children's group, with the parents participating in a 'parent learning' session. Here specific themes are introduced with audio-visual presentations or activities, followed by reflective discussions and mini-role plays. The parallel children's group focuses on improving peer interactions. During the *second hour*, children and parents work together in the same room, with the parents attempting to implement with their children what they have discovered and 'learned' during the first hour. This involves a range of different activities, games and exercises, followed by homework tasks which families can continue the work between MFT sessions.

Each MFT session starts with an *ice-breaker* activity (5–15 minutes) involving all parents and children together. Examples: all family members making a concerted effort to keep soap bubbles in the air, exploring 'how are you feeling?' via Emojis or pictograms, conducting a chorus/orchestra, putting families together with colours of belonging, using string to connect family members with each other. Each session also ends with a joint ritualized parent–child activity, like the previous, which should be the same on every occasion for at least the first four sessions. After the initial ice-breaker activity, the parents leave the larger group room, and the children remain there. The separation process can be videotaped, and the videos can be used as a reviewing tool. Some of the children are likely to find it difficult to actively participate in MFT activities and may instead remain preoccupied with a toy/object or with a self-centred activity. This allows parents to consider how to manage non-participation and to come up with joint action plans. Parents are also encouraged to film typical difficult interactions that occur at home or in other settings (park, shopping centre, friends, etc.) for subsequent presentation and discussion in the parents' group.

Session 1: An autistic view of the world

Parent learning

Video sequence example (e.g., 'seeing the world through the autistic child's eyes'). Discussion as to how this applies to their own children in terms of both strengths and difficulties and what consequences this has for their ways of managing them.

MFT activity

Each parent–child pair tries to make non-verbal contact with another parent and their child. Parents are encouraged to mirror their child and imitate how the child communicates, adapting their imitation in response to feedback from the child. This is videotaped and reviewed by all.

Session 2: Addressing sensory overstimulation

Parent learning

Video sequence example and discussion. Parents then experiment with how to manage different inputs in all sensory modalities, with their intensity being varied and parents reporting how they are affected. Parents then explore self-calming strategies and try these out in pairs.

MFT activity

Slow increase and decrease of sensory overload via music, new toys and games, with the parents developing their ability to pick up and respond to their child's cues and helping their children to improve their self-calming capacity.

Session 3: How autism affected the family's life

Parent learning

Each parent engages in the *Life River* activity, with a specific focus on when autism entered and became a 'travel companion'. Subsequent speculations are invited on how the life river might have continued if autism had not visited the family.

MFT activity

Single-family tasks involving structured play by each parent in parallel with their child. Focus on early signs of parental frustration when child does not comply and how to manage negative affect and to protect child from it.

Session 4: Managing meltdowns

Parent learning

Video examples of meltdown; these can include videos parents bring. Collection of parental strategies. Beginning of parents writing a 'managing meltdown' manual.

MFT activity

Spaghetti and Marshmallows activity. Parents experimenting with new strategies to prevent or reduce meltdowns of child(ren).

Session 5: Structure, order and predictability

Parent learning

Each parent creates their very own pictogram for typical family structure and rules. Parents view and discuss and adapt pictograms.

MFT activity

Parents show the pictogram to their child, explain it and work with it.

Session 6: Repetitive behaviours and OCD-like tendencies

Parent learning

Video examples of repetitive behaviours. Discussion about the advantages and disadvantages of disrupting repetitive behaviours in different situations.

MFT activity

Focusing on repetitive behaviours and experimenting with breaking rituals.

Session 7: New situations

MFT activity

An outing with all families, going to the park, shopping centre, zoo and so on. Subsequent viewing of video examples in a parent-only session of successful and problematic situations.

Session 8: Self-injurious behaviours

Parent learning

Examples, both on video or reported, of interactions with children when they hurt themselves. Experiences and strategies are collected and discussed.

MFT activity

Bag Towers: each family gets a mat on which their child lies on their abdomen. Parents are asked to slowly put weighting bags on their child's back, who are asked to signal with words their responses, like 'yes', 'no', 'more' or via pictograms. Once completed, the bag towers are compared and the effect on the children is discussed.

3. Coming out of the shell

Overview and format

This intensive MFT project, delivered in specialist services, is suitable for families with children under the age of 3 presenting with severe autism and related neurodevelopmental disorders. It consists of 24 sessions of 3 hours in weekly intervals. The sessions are structured around themes, such as sensory experiences and sensory overload, understanding intentions and affect regulation, behaviour and socialization, spontaneous and facilitated communication, sensory overload, sensations and emotions, sensory adjustments, stigma and self-esteem. The programme incorporates innovative techniques, like augmentative and alternative communication

(AAC), psychomotor rehabilitation, postural control development and sensory integration. It is mostly, but not exclusively, for primary carers who attend Out of the Shell MFT. With two-parent families, the other parent (usually the father) joins a once monthly 2-hour 'parents only' group in the evening to address co-parenting issues.

Once every 2 weeks additional two-family observation sessions take place, lasting 2 hours. Here two parents from different families pair up and focus with one practitioner on the strengths and developmental difficulties of their respective child. Problems and how to manage these are identified and described in simple language, such as 'my child has to take my hand first to make a request of me'. After 6 weeks, each parent develops a formal project with the practitioners, focusing on managing two specific problems, formulating hypotheses which may underlie these problems and identifying objectives and resources to achieve these. Work on these projects is carried out in single-family sessions.

Session structure

09:00 Families arrive and socialize spontaneously, with their children engaging with toys and objects present in the waiting area, prior to entering the room in which MFT takes place.

09:15 The children are engrossed in a free play activity, always in the same playground or room, while the parents talk to about how they managed during the previous week. The parents help each other avoid responding automatically to seemingly inappropriate demands made by their children. In the very first session, standing up in a circle, the parents briefly introduce themselves and their child. The practitioners then hand each parent a sheet of paper with five questions which, as each parent walks from one parent to the next, they require them to answer: '*What is my child's name? How old is he? What may be his favourite activity? What may be his strangest behaviour? What may I feel when I don't understand?*' While the first two questions are likely to have been answered during the introduction, the remaining three encourage mentalizing. This activity can be repeated in some of the subsequent sessions.

09:30 The start-up ritual always happens the group room, with the same song greeting the children one by one. The parents are asked to observe how other parents try to make their children understand them. The focus is on non-verbal communication.

09:45 Children and parents are divided then into two groups which take place in separate rooms. The parents take part in the experiential activity selected in accordance with the theme of the morning. Psychoeducational materials of filmed footage of child–parent interactions can be presented. They may, for example, view video segments showing errors in the interpretation of gestures, sequences of non-verbal communication or sequences where adults imitate the behaviours of autistic children to relate to them. The children participate in work based on the developmental social-pragmatic model (DSP; Binns &Cardy, 2019).

10:30 Break

10:45 Parents put into practice with their children what they worked on during the experiential activity. Cross-fostering may be used on occasion, with the parent watching from behind the one-way mirror or video-link how their child is being managed by another parent. Together the parents determine which parental communications are best understood by children and the co-develop a user-friendly 'communication guide' for understanding and managing children with severe autism.

11:15 Parents reflect in their group and on their observations, via video feedback, mini-role plays or speed-dating with a focus on problem-solving. The children have a snack and a relaxing time with low-level stimulation (hypo-stimulation).

12:45 The ending ritual activity involves the same good-bye song addressing the children one by one, followed by children spending time with their respective parents without the practitioners being present.

12:00 Finish

4. Challenging anorexia nervosa

Overview and format

Some 25 years ago, eating disorder teams in Dresden (Universitätsklinikum Carl Gustav Carus) and London (Maudsley Hospital) started intensive MFT approaches for adolescents suffering from anorexia nervosa (Scholz & Asen, 2001; Dare & Eisler, 2000). These treatment programmes have since been further developed (Simic & Eisler, 2015) and are now much applied in Europe and North America, consisting of 10 to 12 sessions of 7 to 8 hours each, over a period of 6 to 9 months. MFT is often delivered in specialist services which also provide paediatric follow-up, as well as individual and single-family therapy. Several different manuals have been published (see, for example, Simic et al., 2023). MFT eating disorder approaches have also been developed for adults but tend to be less effective, not the least because of the very chronic nature of the illness and the deeply entrenched patterns (Baudinet et al., 2021; Baudinet et al., 2023).

The work starts with a 'tasting event' which takes place a few weeks (and sometimes only a few days) before the start of the formal programme. The aim is to let families have a first experience of what MFT is all about and for them to make last-minute decisions as to whether they want to take part or not. The programme starts with 4 days (Monday to Thursday), from 9.00 to 16.30, followed by another 2 days in a row some 2 weeks later, 2 more days in a row some 3 to 4 weeks later, and the remaining sessions are 1 day each month. All sessions have a fairly similar structure (see Box 8).

Box 8   Structure of day

9:00   informal welcome of families, storage of meals they have brought and weighing of young people
9:30   ice-breaker and single-family activities
10:30   morning snack
11:00   second activity
12:30   joint meal, followed by a 30-minute break
13:45   third activity
15:15   afternoon snack
15:45   final activity and discussion of transfer task
16:30   end of session

The three mealtimes during each session are of central importance, as problematic eating and feeding patterns emerge naturally and can be observed by everyone as the families sit all at the same large table. The practitioners witness the stress experienced by the adolescents as well as by their parents, and these permit practitioners to consider making specific interventions. The joint mealtimes also provide opportunities for families to observe each other and work together to challenge anorectic eating dynamics.

Session overview

Session 1: Tasting event

The 3-hour evening begins with a formal presentation of MFT, its concepts and effectiveness. This is followed by a series of ice-breaker activities (e.g., *Catch the Ball, Speed-Dating*); a collaborative psychoeducation meeting is then convened with the families being invited to list everything they know about anorexia nervosa. Families then meet 'graduate families', which allows questions about MFT to be answered by 'experts by experience'. During the last part of the tasting event, small sub-groups are formed, with members of different families talking to each other and reflecting about what they have heard and experienced. Up to 15 families may attend a tasting event, and if they all subsequently decide to participate in the MFT programme, two parallel groups may start at the same time if there are sufficient practitioners available. Alternatively, a waiting list group may need to be formed, as the maximum number of families should not exceed six or seven.

Session 2: Getting to know anorexia

Activity 1: The session starts with the *Geography Sculpt*.

Activity 2: The families interview each other in pairs about their expectations and fears. They can be given three specific questions and have to imagine that they are journalists when posing these. Typical questions are: '*When did anorexia first visit your family and what happened?*'; '*What fears, if any, do you have about attending MFT?*'; '*What are each family member's hopes?*' Having collected the answers to these questions and written these on a journalist's notepad, families interview each other in turn. When the process is finished (after 10–20 minutes), the large group is reconvened, and each family introduces briefly the family they had interviewed to the group: '*This is the Smith family and anorexia first turned up when . . .*'. This is followed by a snack (15 minutes) with the families all sitting around a large table, with their adolescent child next to them. It is the first (small) meal of the day, and the practitioners only observe the emerging interaction patterns around food, 'bookmarking' these without intervening.

Activity 3: Each adolescent is asked to draw a *Portrait of Anorexia* while the parents work on their meal targets for the week ahead, exchanging ideas. This is followed by the main meal (45 minutes) and then 15 minutes of unstructured time.

Activity 3: The parents share their experiences of the first observed mealtime while the adolescents stage an exhibition with the anorexia portraits. The parents visit the exhibition and are formally interviewed by journalists, the adolescents, about their impressions, thoughts and feelings about each portrait.

Activity 4: The *Affect Snapshots* taken during to the day are viewed on a screen/laptop and group members are encouraged to speculate about mental states displayed.

Session 3: Managing eating dynamics

The session starts with an icebreaker activity (e.g., *Finding your Place*).

Activity 1: The group is divided into adults and adolescents, and a festive meal is prepared for each family. The adolescents compose the meal they think their parents might want to make for them on a special occasion. Meanwhile, in another part of the room, each set of parents composes the actual meal they would want to give their child on the special occasion. The meals are made of collages of food images and are placed on cardboard plates. Parents and adolescents then compare their prepared meals.

Activity 2: In a role play, the adolescents, pretending to be their parents, try to convince their parents, pretending to be their adolescent children, to eat the symbolic meals. The parents, in the role of their children, are asked to use all the sentences and words their children tend to use when they refuse to eat. There is likely to be a lot of laughter, and after each family has finished, they can exchange their experiences with others.

Activity 3: The adolescents are cross-fostered during the (real) lunch, with each adolescent sitting next to the parents of another adolescent. Once lunchtime is over, the parents discuss their experiences in a fishbowl scenario, with the adolescents placed in 'outside' listening positions. This is then reversed, with the parents listening to the adolescents' debriefing.

Activity 4: Relaxation and mindfulness exercises are introduced, and families are encouraged to practice these.

Session 4: The impact of the illness on family relationships

Siblings are invited to this session which starts with an icebreaker activity, like keeping soap bubbles in the air, a task requiring much collaboration. This can be set up as a competition between families.

Activity 1: Adolescents and siblings form a group and engage in one of the following activities: *Family Crest/or Family Website.* In a separate group, the parents are exposed to statements projected on a large screen (e.g., '*Until something clicks in my child's head, they won't be able to get better despite our help*', '*When it comes to caring for our sick child, it's best to leave our brothers and sisters alone so as not to worry them,* '*It's not always advisable to be firm with a child who has anorexia, as this can hurt them or make them suffer too much*'). With each statement, the parents are asked to position themselves spatially according to their level of agreement by moving closer to the screen or further away. They then engage in a discussion about their different points of view.

Activity 2: Live Sculpting. A sculptor is appointed in each family, with the task of placing the members of their family and themselves in such a way as to represent their current relationships. 'Anorexia' is then added to the sculpt, represented by a masked practitioner.

Activity 3: A special sibling workshop is held with the theme 'What we think about anorexia'. In a separate group, each anorectic adolescent writes two letters to the anorectic young person ('*Dear Jane, anorexia loves you because . . .* ' and '*Dear Jane, anorexia hates you because . . .* '). In parallel, the parents prepare a role play on '*Tricks anorexia plays in the family*'.

Activity 4: Presentation of the work the siblings completed. This can be done in the form of a mock TV show.

Session 5: Family strengths and support

Icebreaker: Body Feelings.

Activity 1: The adolescents and their fathers do the *Blind Trust* activity. The mothers in parallel draw up the Job Descriptions and *Job References* for mothers of anorectic teenagers. Where the family consists of same-sex or single parents, the family decides who should do what. If a family thinks that it is more appropriate for the mother to do the *Blind Trust* activity and the father to do the job description activity, that is fine.

Activity 2: The female adolescents and their mothers participate in the *Body Image Poster* activity. (Male adolescents can do this with their fathers.) In parallel, the fathers discuss their role as 'second line' helpers supporting the mothers, who tend to be on the 'front line'. This redefines their role in functional terms rather than stigmatizing the fathers' seeming 'distance'. In some families these more traditional gender roles will not apply. This can be explored and different views and experiences shared.

Activity 3: The adolescents construct an Anorexia First Aid Kit, accompanied by a written instructions for parents. In parallel, the parents design a *Survival Manual in the Land of Anorexia*. When the two sub-groups join, the written instructions for parents are read out by the adolescents.

Activity 4: The practitioners form a reflective team in a fishbowl setting, commenting on the observations they have made over the first 4 days.

Session 6: Understanding feeling states

Activity 1: In separate groups (one with parents, one with adolescents) one, two or three positive events and one, two or three difficult events that occurred over the previous fortnight are identified. A *newspaper headline* for each event is created, and, when the two groups meet, each side has to guess what the headlines refer to.

Activity 2: The adolescents define the advantages (everything that anorexia forces them to do and what anorexia does for them) and the disadvantages of having anorexia (everything that anorexia prevents them from doing and what anorexia does for them) in their lives. In parallel to this activity, the parents put on a large weighing scale the actions and attitudes that, in their view, motivate the adolescent to get better and those that encourage them to stay ill.

Activity 3: All group members participate in the *Mind Scan* activity. They are told that a new medical imaging tool has been developed which permits scanning people's minds. Each family member is appointed to be a mentalizing radiologist and fill in the brain diagram (see Chapter 6), speculating what might be going on in the mind of each family member. The images are then formally presented by the 'radiologists' and comments and reflections are invited.

Activity 4: Traps and Treasures: The practitioners state that the (seeming) *benefits* of anorexia as seen by the adolescents have become *traps*, and that the *drawbacks* have become *treasures*. Treasures are small pieces of paper on which situations are written that anorexia prevents adolescents from doing (e.g., *'going to the cinema'*, *'going out with the family'*). Traps are small pieces of paper, stuck to noisy obstacles, which contain situations that anorexia forces people to do (e.g., *'counting calories'*, *'arguing with each other'*). An obstacle course is set up and the adolescents guide their blindfolded parents through the course, avoiding the traps and collecting the treasures. The roles are then reversed. After three rounds or more, each family finds out which treasures they have won and which traps they have avoided.

Session 7: Managing emotions and conflicts

Siblings are invited to attend this session.

Activity 1: Each family participates in the *Spaghetti and Marshmallows* activity.

Activity 2: In parallel, parents' and children's groups do the *Care Tags* activity.

Activity 3: Slow *Speed-Dating* involving all group members to reflect on the different care tags.

Session 8: Managing uncertainty

The session starts with an icebreaker activity (e.g., *Who has ever . . . ?)*

Activity 1: Each family draws a *Family Network Map*, which, once completed, is presented to the other families.

Activity 2: The adolescents participate in a 5 Senses Workshop (discovering food through hearing, smelling, looking, touching and tasting, both individually and together). In parallel, the parents take part in an activity called *moving for-ward with composure in an uncertain world*. The room is divided into four areas along two axes (safe/unsafe and certainty/uncertainty), and the parents position themselves according to their own experiences of when change threatened (e.g., moving house, changing jobs, welcoming their in-laws). They are then asked to consider their respective children and how they might place themselves in relation to change (e.g., first day at a new school, closing a social media account, having to tell a friend that they have hurt their feelings). The parents then discuss together what enabled them to manage these situations.

Activity 3: Each family participates in the *Family Timelines* activity.

Activity 4: All group members participate in the *Lie Detector* activity.

Session 9: Calling on one's relational resources

Grandparents, aunts, uncles and family friends are invited to this session.

Activity 1: The parents meet with the various relatives and collect questions they would like to have answered. In parallel, the adolescents prepare answers to the likely questions for the press.

Activity 2: Press Conference.

Activity 3: Small sub-groups are formed with the task to define how relatives can be helpful for the adolescent and the family. The adolescents then each write a letter to 'dear relatives', providing ideas how they can be helpful and not, that is, specifying dos and don'ts for family and friends.

Session 10: Self-empowerment

Activity 1: Adolescents are invited to take part in the *Cost-Effective* Dances activity. Parents are invited to guide and accompany their child during a dance that should bring serenity and economy (a calorimeter is placed in the adolescent's pocket). The parents are not allowed to touch their child.

Activity 2: Each family does the *Life River* activity.

Activity 3: The fathers and adolescents build a *Survival Suitcase*. In parallel, the mothers reflect on what their adolescent children expect and need in terms of autonomy and what they can do to support it.

Activity 4: Mothers and adolescents engage in the *Wellness Farm* activity. In parallel, the fathers on what their adolescent children expect and need in terms of autonomy and what they can do to support it. As with other activities, same-sex and single-parent families can make decisions themselves regarding how they engage, as can families who feel strongly that traditional gender roles are not applicable to them.

Session 11: Looking ahead and relapse prevention

Activity 1: Masked Ball.

Activity 2: A case presentation. The case of a young person who is in recovery but has to leave home to study is presented to the families. The adolescents are asked to mentalize their parents' expectations and fears, and the parents mentalize the young person's expectations and fears. A role play debate is then organized, with the parents (playing the young person) asking the parents (played by the adolescents) what guarantees they give the young person in terms of autonomy if they have to stay at home. The adolescents in turn question the parents (playing the young person) to find out what guarantees the young person can give them in terms of safety.

Activity 3: 'Everything you always wanted to know about adolescence but were afraid to ask'. In this enactment, the parents are the experts on their own adolescence and are interviewed by the adolescents who are acting as journalists.

Activity 4: The families meet without the practitioners to decide on the structure of the final session.

Session 12: Ending and planning the future

The entire day is organized and run by the families themselves. The practitioners are merely in an observing position, refusing to give any guidance or advice.

5. Breaking taboos – MFT for bulimia nervosa

Overview and format

This project for bulimia nervosa and binge eating disorders is designed for adolescents between the ages of 12 to18 years. It consists of 14 weekly sessions of 2 hours each. The first session is attended by both the adolescents and their parents. Sessions 2 to 5 are split: after a short ice-breaker activity, parents and young people work in separate groups so that the teenagers can talk about their difficulties without shame and develop a shared understanding of the problem. On the parents' side, the aim is to reduce hostility and to help them mentalize their young person's needs and to experience empathic validation. In session 6, the young people first devise a presentation and then present their work to the parents. Sessions 7 to 14 are joint sessions with both parents and adolescents, focusing on both relaxation and themed activities.

The content of the project is based on the typical cycle of emotional regulation one finds in young people suffering from bulimia nervosa (Byrne & McLean, 2002): anxiety > binge eating > guilt > purging > shame > hiding > conflict > loneliness > insecurity. Parents respond with their cycle of anxiety: helplessness > hypervigilance > conflict > hostility > lack of confidence > anxiety. These connected and resonating cycles define the themes of work with this group of families.

Session 1: Tasting event

Families are welcomed with refreshments and are then given a formal presentation of the MFT and its theory and practice. This is followed by *Speed Dating*, with the adolescents in the inner and the parents in the outer circle. The focus of some of the questions is on the expectations and hopes and fears everyone has. These are subsequently collected by the practitioners when they interview group members about what they have heard from others. Small groups are randomly assigned, and each group shares their experiences and familiarizes themselves with the concept of a cycle which bulimia nervosa triggers. They can talk about the individual characteristics (people's thoughts, behaviours, emotions) and the interactions and situations which contribute to this 'odd cycle'. If group members are having difficulty coming up with ideas, they can consult a 'black box', placed in the middle of the room which contains descriptions of the binge-purge cycle and the conflict-avoidance relationship cycle. Each group then reports what they themselves have found out about the 'odd cycle'. Towards the end of the tasting event, the rules for the group are discussed and agreed, in the form of a 'MFT Group Constitution'.

Session 2: On emotional rollercoasters

Sessions 2 to 5 – each session begins with an ice-breaker, such as the *Catch The Ball* or *Finding Your Place*, Finding Your Place. The rest of the session takes place in split groups, with the parents on one side and adolescents on the other.

After the initial icebreaker, a *Slow Speed Dating* invites all group members to talk about any thoughts and feelings they had during or after the tasting event. During the speed dating, the practitioners take photographs (*Affect Snapshots*) of everyone. The group is then divided into two: one for the adolescents, the other for the parents.

- Adolescents: postcards and photos of people (but *not* of the group participants) are presented, and group members are invited to speculate about the mental states depicted, as well as discussing their beliefs about emotions and their effect on thoughts and behaviours. If the practitioners find it relevant and possible, they propose further work, using the snapshots of the parents.

- Parents: in sub-groups of three or four, the parents discuss the impact of bulimia nervosa on family relationships. They are then asked to provide examples of problematic interaction sequences involving bulimic dynamics, and these are then staged in the form of a role play. Each phase of the evolving interaction is 'frozen', and the observing are invited to reflect on the effects on the parent's mental states, triggered by their interactions with their child.

Session 3: Managing distress

The group is divided into two: one for the adolescents, the other for the parents.

- Adolescents: Videos of stressful situations are presented, like receiving an upsetting phone message, arriving in the crowd of a new high school during the start of the school year or a young person being bullied. The evoked emotions and how one has managed to contain them, or not, are discussed in pairs. The adolescents relay appropriate and inappropriate affect management strategies.
- Parents: In groups of two, the parents watch a video sequence depicting meal interactions between a child and a parent. They are asked to speculate about the emotional state of the child and the parent. They then consider what else could have been done at each phase during the evolving interactions, taking into account the likely emotional needs of each of the protagonists. The parents are then presented with the affect snapshots that had been taken of their children during the second session.

Session 4: To validate or not to validate

The group is divided into two: one for the adolescents, the other for the parents.

- Adolescents: Collaborative psychoeducation is used to explore the concept of an emotional regulation cycle involving hyperphagic binges and compensatory behaviours – purging, restriction and hyperactivity. The advantages and disadvantages of such a cycle are discussed. Each teenager creates their own cycle and discusses it with the other young people.
- Parents: A role play is set up, with one parent confiding their difficulties to another who is asked to minimize and trivialize these. This is done in a fishbowl setting, with the other parents watching the role plays and then reflecting how this is and has been affecting them. The concept of validation is addressed during a collaborative psychoeducation session, with the question: '*does validating mean agreeing?*' The parents then discuss in a *Speed Dating* how and when to validate their child's potentially problematic behaviours – and when not.

Session 5: Breaking out of a dangerously useful cycle

The group is divided into two: one for the adolescents, the other for the parents.

- Adolescents: in a group, the adolescents sketch a 'general hyperphagia/compensation cycle' (*not* one of any young person present!). In sub-groups, they identify the factors that influence it and add them to their presentation. They choose how to present the cycle in the form of a poster, video, PowerPoint or conference talk.
- Parents: In sub-groups, the parents identify three problematic situations which they act out in brief role plays. The observers of the role plays are asked to speculate about the young persons' mental states and suggest helpful validation statements. The role-played adolescents are asked in role about how the validation statements affected them. The parents then discuss their difficulties with producing authentic validation statements in pairs and try to compose new and better fitting ones.

Session 6: Presentation of the hyperphagia/compensation cycle

The session starts with a 15-minute relaxation or mindfulness activity. The adolescents then present their work on the hyperphagia/compensation cycle. They are encouraged to be as didactic as possible. Parents are encouraged to ask exploratory questions and be curious about aspects of the presentation. Reflective time is staged in a 'foster family' setting, discussing the advantages of considering their problems from the perspective of this cycle. At the end of the session, each family is assigned the responsibility of finding and leading a mindfulness/relaxation activity for one of the subsequent sessions.

Session 7: Identifying and managing emotions

Sessions 7 to 14: Each session begins with a 10- to 15-minute mindfulness/relaxation activity led by a different family each time. During all these sessions, the poster/work on the overeating/compensation cycle is displayed prominently in the room.

All adolescents are cross-fostered and the 'foster parents' support them doing the *Body Feelings* activity. The posters are hung up on the wall and subgroups of peers go from poster to poster and propose ideas for self-regulation on Post-Its. At a later stage, the families recompose into the original family and exchange with them the ideas presented on the Post-Its. At the end of this session, each family is asked to bring a small survival kit back to the next session.

Session 8: Managing crises

Parents and children identify problematic situations between them. A possible scenario can be introduced by the practitioners, such as '*The parents have arranged a dinner party, the guests arrive and the parents realize that all the chips and the desert have been devoured, they go to see the young person*' and played out. Group members then mentalize in small groups of two or three the psychological states of the parents and adolescents and identify any mentalizing blocks. They then work on looking for alternatives which they replay (rewriting scenarios) to evaluate the effects. They write down these alternatives on cards, and each family chooses which ones to take in the first aid kit they have purchased. An alternative is to use the *Escalation Clock* activity.

Session 9: Managing social relationships

Families do the *Circle Game* activity and then think about the advantages and disadvantages of social relationships during speed dating. Then, divided into small groups, parents and adults identify the repercussions of social relationships on emotions and thoughts. The subgroups then work on individual tools for managing emotions and thoughts in relationships. Three metaphors are introduced: the 'strainer', which allows one to filter what one wants to take into a relationship and what one wants to leave behind; the 'buzzer', which allows one to exit a situation before emotions and thoughts become overloaded; and the 'thermostat', which permits one not to be overwhelmed by strong emotions. They write survival techniques and tools on cards for each the 'strainer', 'buzzer' and 'thermostat' (e.g., '*in this case . . . do . . .* '). Each family then decides which tools they will fill the young person's first aid kit with.

Session 10: Asking for help and developing trust

During this session, the *Blind Trust* activity is introduced, and then parents think in pairs about ways to ask for help and support when one is in difficulty and feels ashamed and guilty. The adolescents think about how to deliver help and support so that they can accept it. Each family then focuses on a transfer task: finding a situation of moderate difficulty during which help and support will be provided.

Session 11: Using family resources

The main activity of this session is *Live Sculptures*. Each family prepares a sculpture of how their members perceive current family relationships. They then present their sculpture to other families who associate, mentalize and comment freely. Solutions can be brainstormed between group members if a family situation appears particularly blocked. Then each family is led to make their sculpture of the future and then to imagine the individual and relational steps that must be taken to achieve this.

Session 12: Identifying resources in difficult situations

Each family is invited to carry out the *Life River* activity. Once finished, these are presented to each other, and comments and questions are invited. Subsequent work in subgroups aims to identify the resources that made it possible to overcome/adapt to life's obstacles.

Session 13: Achieving autonomy

Each family carries out the *Survival Suitcase* activity. The parents and children reflect on values and resources to become independent and avoid relapses. Then the families meet without the practitioners to decide on the themes and activities they wish to carry out for their last session.

Session 14: Do it yourselves . . .

Families organize this session, with the practitioners in the backseat.

6. Managing suicidal and self-harming adolescents

Overview and format

This hospital-based programme, for adolescents aged 12 to 18 and their families, aims to reduce the risk of suicide and self-harm. The eight sessions last 3 hours, with the first three spaced one week apart and sessions 4 to 8 then taking place fortnightly. The group structure outlined in the following can be varied in response to expectations and themes families bring during the first session.

Session overview

Session 1: Tasting event

Families are welcomed, and a formal presentation of the objectives, principles, framework and process of MFT is provided. This is followed by speed-dating, with questions focusing on hobbies, the characteristics of family members and what worries family members the most. In parallel groups, parents and adolescents explore each other's expectations, listing them and regrouping them. Parents and children then get together and try to guess what each group has come up with. Parents and adolescents then share their expectations and rank the most important themes. Parents and children then work separately on the group rules before pooling their ideas around the theme: how can safety be ensured in the group?

Session 2: Ensuring safety

The session is started with two icebreakers, like every group member calling out their names and each family keeping soap bubbles as long in the air as possible. Families then think about how one can cooperate if one has to take care of something fragile. The next activity consists of watching a video of a family argument between a mother and her adolescent from a fictional film. Group members are invited to mentalize the protagonists and develop interventions to achieve different outcomes. Group members are then asked to describe typical crisis situations involving their young person. Based on the example, role plays involving risk-taking are set up (e.g., young person suddenly leaves and locks themselves in their room). Parents begin to create a manual depicting prevention plans for various scenarios.

Session 3: Externalizing the problems

Siblings are invited to attend. Icebreaker activity: *Who has Ever...?* The parents and young persons are then separated into two groups. The latter are invited to talk about their problems and specify the following: Is the problem small or big? What impact does it have on you? What are their aims/goals and how might they achieve these? For their part, the parents list the problems they identify in their young people, as well as the early signs of these problems emerging, and then reflect on the impact that the problem has on them. The siblings have the same task, but in a separate group. The groups then come together and share their reflections in small sub-groups. This is followed by the *Live Sculpture* activity, with each family representing their relationships around the problem. Group members are asked to discuss during each family sculpture, what they identify as the emotions, mindsets and relationships that maintain the problem and the emotions, mindsets and relationships that are evidence of family strengths. Each family then thinks about how they can employ their strengths and resources to decrease the impact of the problem.

Session 4: Identifying affect

The session starts with the activity *How Others See You*, followed by a reflective round about anxieties relating to what other people think about oneself. This is followed by the adolescents participating in the *Body Feelings* activity, with a subsequent discussion on the different manifestations of feelings first and then on the strategies one can put in place to regulate them. In their own group, the parents participate in the *Affect Snapshots* activity, focusing on the adolescents' faces and their possible states of mind. They are invited to speculate about 'problematic' and 'functional' examples of affect and relate these to past situations and how they did respond to each 'face' – and how one might respond differently in the future. The parents are asked to then imagine the adolescents' needs in different scenarios. The adolescents then curate an exhibition of their *Body Feelings* images, guiding their parents from poster to poster and inviting their reflections. The focus is on how to identify and regulate complex emotions and this is afterwards discussed in small sub-groups. Examples of relaxation and mindfulness exercises are invited and/or demonstrated.

Session 5: Managing emotional crises

The session is started with the *Blind Trust* activity, followed by reflections in random sub-groups on issues of trust – when it is justified and when it is misplaced.

This is followed by each adolescent being 'cross-fostered' (see Chapter 3) with the 'foster parent' interviewing the young person to understand the dynamics of the crisis: its level of intensity, its evolutionary mode (initial phase, peak, decline) and the factors which influence it. The trajectory of the crisis is drawn as a 'crisis curve' by each parent for their child. The parents then discuss what they have discovered about the respective crises and try to find ways of intervening before, during and after the crisis, as well as considering the factors which influence it. During this time, the young people do the *Care Tags* activity. This is followed by speed-dating, with the parents (in the outer circle) finding out about the needs of the adolescents (in the inner circle). After that, each family examines the specific crisis curve the parent has drawn and considers one of the young person's needs and how this can be met between sessions.

Session 6: Communicating about dark thoughts and feelings

The central activity of the session is the *Press Conference*. The adolescents, in their own group, prepare expert responses on how to manage suicidal crises. They may collect the relevant information via collaborative psychoeducation and using testimonies from 'survivors'. The parents, in their parallel group, prepare questions which, in their role as 'journalists', they will ask the 'experts'. After the press conference, the parents, in their group, are encouraged to reflect on what they have learned from their children and to consider whether they view their respective child differently, having heard their contributions during the press conference. The young people, in their group, reflect on the necessary conditions and circumstances to permit good and appropriate communication between parents and children about suicidal crises to take place and considering the advantages and disadvantages of talking with their parents about these.

Session 7: Relapse prevention

Each family starts the session by doing the *Life River* activity. The different diagrams are presented, and in the discussions the focus is on how to overcome the obstacles and vicissitudes of life. This is followed by randomly divided subgroups in which members identify all the concrete ways that make it possible to face difficult times. These are documented on a piece of paper and read out once the large group has reconvened. Each family then chooses some of the ideas to compose an 'adolescent's first-aid kit'. During the last part of the session, families are asked to plan how to structure the last session and to think about and devise a parting ritual.

Session 8: Parting and moving on . . .

The families implement the structure and content they developed during the last session. Time is set aside for the parting ritual.

7. Working with psychosis

Overview

MFT for families containing a person with schizophrenia or other forms of psychosis goes back right to the birth and early development of the approach (Laqueur et al., 1964; McFarlane et al., 1993). Psychoeducational in essence, a major aim of the work is to increase the families' coping skills in managing symptoms and prevent relapse, partly by reducing the key relatives' levels of expressed emotion (EE), and above all the critical comments and over-involvement (Vaughn & Leff, 1976). The hypothesis is that families containing a psychotic member develop dysfunctional and 'counterintuitive' strategies and therefore need to be taught more functional ones (McFarlane et al., 1993), being 'taught' what they do not 'know' and therefore developing ways of dealing with positive and negative symptoms, often by painful trial and error. The approach also focuses on reducing caregiver burden, that is, the stress and strain a caregiver experiences as a result of caring for a family member who is chronically ill. The demands of caregiving can be exhausting and overwhelming. The psychoeducational approach holds that families containing a person with psychosis need to possess all the available knowledge about the illness and the treating practitioners are seen as the major source of that information. Another major emphasis of the approach is on problem solving, such as dealing with aggressive and suicidal behaviours; managing family conflicts, ensuring compliance with medication and medical advice and controlling substance and alcohol misuse. A specific problem is selected for each MFT session, and the group members are encouraged to list possible solutions and discussing the advantages and disadvantages of each in turn. Finally, the solution that best fits the situation is agreed upon and a detailed implementation plan is developed (McFarlane et al 1993). McFarlane's and his colleagues' work is well researched and has a solid evidence base (see also Chapter 2). However, it has only partly informed the systemic MFT approach put forward in this book, as there are some significant differences, above all the focus on activating the families' resources and to elicit their own, often buried, knowledge and 'know-how'. With the help of the Internet, books, newspapers, journals and other publications, families are now in a different position to have access to potentially relevant information than was the case a few decades ago. Systemic MFT relies a lot on families inspiring and 'psycho-educating' each other.

Prior to starting MFT, families with psychotic members require some preparation. This can take the form of meeting with each family on their own on two or three occasions, ideally in the presence of a professional from the local community mental health team who is already connected with the family. These single-family meetings promote understanding of the issues each family is struggling with and help the family members to feel listened to and understood. It is our experience that engagement in subsequent MFT work is significantly increased via these initial encounters, and non-attendance or early drop-out rates are reduced (Asen & Schuff, 2006). The work can then be started with an initial whole-day 'workshop'. This term emphasizes the collaborative nature of the day, which is very structured, with two-way presentations on specific themes (e.g., stigma, medication compliance, double diagnosis issues), followed by small group discussions. Informal socializing takes place over lunch, followed by a multifamily activity (e.g., *Letter to the Problem*), and the workshop is concluded with a final plenary, when families list what they have discovered during the workshop. This first day is followed by 2-hour MFT sessions at fortnightly or three-weekly intervals.

Group membership does not need to be restricted to one particular diagnostic category, as the differences between conditions, such as schizophrenia, bipolar or schizoaffective illness, are not all that marked when it comes to considering the common problems for families of having to cope with radical changes in their lives. Flexibility is important, and families should be able to bring new members or friends to the group or invite a trusted professional, for example, their community psychiatric nurse or their social worker. Groups can be closed or semi-open, depending on the context within which they take place: in mental hospitals, for example, it may make sense to have a semi-open group, with new families entering the project when others leave.

Systemic MFT lends itself particularly to working with families in the early stages of a psychotic disorder, as family members then tend to be centrally involved and still more open to participation. This effectively means working with adolescents and younger adults. Acutely psychotic patients are difficult to contain in MFT, and if or when they relapse, they will not attend MFT until their mental states are more settled. When attempting to adapt this model to the work with chronic and institutionalized in-patients, it tends to be more difficult to activate relatives who often have, many years ago, handed over all the care of their ill family members to mental hospital staff.

The MFT sessions consist of whole-group discussions when positive and negative experiences are shared. A wide range of topics and issues is covered, and it is useful to focus on one theme for each session, as described in the following case example. Multifamily activities should be part of each session so that too much repetitive talking does not prevail. These can include *Body Feelings, Clay Family Sculptures, Mood Barometer* or *Letters to the Illness*.

It is very important for MFT projects to be embedded in the wider service context even though the model supports the notion that the family is – or becomes – the main care provider. Local community mental health teams (CMHTs) are very frequently involved, and as MFT fosters collaborative and transparent interactions and communications among professionals, patients and their carers, group members are encouraged to use their respective psychiatric services as well, to have more of a say with regard to service provision and the shaping of 'their' treatments.

MFT with this group of families can be challenging. For example, if one group member – a relative or a patient – dominates the meeting, it is usually much easier for a member of staff to create appropriate boundaries than it is for other members of the group. On other occasions, a person with psychosis might become overwhelmed or confused by the group process: the practitioner will then need to create appropriate min-contexts to lower the quantity of stimuli and emotion. This can lead to setting up a brief small sub-group which allows space for the affected person. Staff may occasionally need to protect unwell individuals from being exposed to high EE comments and interactions from one of their relatives or from members of other families. However, this is, in our experience, a rare event, as multi-family groups develop their own rules of 'good conduct'.

Format

A project can take six to eight families containing a psychotic member, age 16 to 25. Single-family preparation takes place first, followed by attendance at a tasting evening. The work starts with a whole-day workshop, followed by 2-hour sessions in fortnightly and then 3-weekly intervals over 1 year. Each of these sessions has a theme which provides the main focus, as described subsequently. Further themes can be added subsequently. When a family member presents with a psychotic episode, their participation will be temporarily suspended until their mental state is stabilized. However, the key relatives can continue to attend the group.

Session overview

Session 1: Whole-day workshop

10.00 Families arrive and socialize
10.30 Collaborative psychoeducation session on psychosis and diagnoses, voices' groups, alternative therapies, expressed emotion, the impact of hospital admission on the family
11.30 Small topic-based group discussion on the previous themes
12.00 Reflections plenary and mid-workshop evaluation
12.30 Joint lunch
13.30 MFT activity: *Family Clay Sculpts* – followed by discussion on how the sculpt would have looked like before psychosis visited the family – and how people think it might look like in 1 year's time
15.00 Tea/coffee break, families socialize
15.30 Problem-Solving Session. Group members agree on three common problems they encounter in relation to psychosis and then work out how to manage each of them. This is done in sub-groups
16.30 Reflections plenary and end-workshop evaluation
17.00 Finish

Themes for subsequent sessions

All sessions have a similar structure. They start with an icebreaker (e.g., speed-dating):

Session 2 The illness, its course and typical crises
Session 3 Medication adherence, alcohol and substance misuse
Session 4 Separation issues and leaving home
Session 5 Partners and friendship issues
Session 6 Parental concerns regarding intrusiveness and over-protection
Session 7 Reducing expressed emotion
Session 8 To work or not to work?
Session 9 Managing strong emotions
Session 10 Involving the social network
Session 11 Limit setting
Session 12 Early relapse signs and relapse prevention

8. Waiting-list MFT

Many child and adolescent mental health services (CAMHS) are overloaded with new referrals, and, as a result, families usually have to wait many months for an initial appointment. Offering MFT groups for these families has proved one way of addressing excessive waiting times. After a brief triage process carried out by a CAMHS professional, families are allocated to a MFT waiting list group which consists of four to eight weekly or fortnightly sessions, each lasting 2 hours. This permits professionals to both offer a quick response, so often requested by parents, as well as observing children and parents in an interactive environment and identifying specific parenting skills and difficulties, as well as assessing children informally and contributing to formulations and diagnoses. The project described in the following is one example of behaviour-focused MFT.

Waiting-list project 'problem behaviours'

Overview

This project consists of eight sessions of 2 hours in weekly intervals, aimed at families with a child, age 6–11, presenting with behavioural difficulties, such as being oppositional defiant, impulsive or easily frustrated and angry.

Session 1: We don't listen to each other!

The session is started with the *Catch the Ball* activity so that families get to know each other. This is followed by the *Remote Control* activity. Each family experiments with their own child. This is then reversed, and the children attempt to remote control their parent(s). Once everyone has had a go, separate parents' and a children's groups are formed, both with the same task: to create the five buttons that would improve family life. The adults and children then compare their respective remote controls, and each family agrees on three buttons they are going to use between this and the next session.

Session 2: Concentrate!

Families are welcomed and take part in the *Who Has Ever....?* activity. Each parent and their child then engage in building a Lego structure. Both parent and child sit at a table opposite each other, and each has a set of Lego pieces. There is a little wall between them, made out of books standing up, so that neither party can see the emerging structure on the other side. Each parent starts building their own structure and tells their child what the colour and shape of the Lego piece is and how it is positioned. As the child cannot see what the parent is building, they need to concentrate and listen carefully, as they can only rely on what they hear when they try to replicate the – to them invisible – structure their parent is building. After 3 minutes, the book-wall is lifted, and parent and child compare their respective structures and discuss similarities and differences – and how these might be explained. The roles are then reversed, with the children instructing their parents in building new constructions. During this activity, the practitioners try to distract parents and children (with sound, light and gestures), to interfere with the participants' concentration. This is followed by the children being 'cross-fostered' and identifying techniques which helped to concentrate. Families are then instructed to repeat the activity and practice new concentration techniques.

Session 3: What excitement!

The session is started with *Speed Dating* when group members find out how the previous week has been for everyone. This is followed by the activity *Popping Balloons*: each child has a balloon tied to their ankle and must burst as many balloons of other children while protecting their own. After 5 minutes of excitement all round, there is then a very fast transition to focusing on a task (a game requiring intense concentration or a math test), which requires downregulating one's arousal. Parents are encouraged to help their child calm down and complete the task. This is followed by a collaborative psychoeducation workshop, focusing on the bodily manifestations of arousal and how to regulate these.

Session 4: A question of trust!

Families gather around a snack to discuss any developments since the previous session. Parents and children participate in the *Blind Trust* activity, taking it in turn to guide each other. Afterwards, in small randomly assigned subgroups, group members identify the best ways to help and guide someone who is having behavioural difficulties.

Session 5: Daily volcano eruptions!

Group members identify everyday situations that pose a problem (e.g., going to bed, stopping video games, not liking the food, getting up and getting ready for school, doing homework, being on their mobile phones all the time). Typical scenarios are role played with a reversal of roles. Specific scenes are 'frozen', and group members are requested to mentalize the states of mind of the protagonists. A reflective time follows on how to spot and prevent future eruptions.

Session 6: Who is the best?

Each child is 'cross-fostered' and joins in fairly quick succession several tables with educational games that require concentration, such as Simon Says, jigsaw puzzles, battleships, checkers, traffic lights. Every 5 minutes, children rotate. This is followed by the *Amoeba Game*. The subsequent reflection time focuses on the themes of sharing moments of being silly, as well as on issues to do with winning, losing and cheating.

Session 7: Family strengths!

In the previous session each family was asked to select 10 photographs that tell the story of their current family and families of origin. Each family creates a *Family Website* with the help of the photos, using felt-tip pens, glue and scissors. The families then present their work to each other and invite comments and questions. Afterwards, children and parents are divided into two separate groups, and each is asked to draw one strength that they believe they received from their family.

Session 8: What a super team!

The group starts with an icebreaker. Following this, families play together a video escape action game and then identify in small groups the ingredients for good cooperation. At the end of the activity, randomly assigned subgroups have the task of identifying the ingredients needed for good collaboration. Families are then asked to provide feedback about the waiting-list MFT project, and professionals can update their initial assessment based on their understanding of the families' needs following the group.

Waiting-list groups for children presenting with other difficulties, for example, those with predominantly emotional symptoms, can take a similar format to the previous one, with the content tailored to meet the specific needs of the group.

Chapter 9

MFT projects in social services settings

Child protection and MFT

One major role of social services departments working with children and families is to ensure young people are safe, looked-after and protected from suffering any form of abuse and neglect. Social services are a key component of child protection systems, and to effectively protect the vulnerable, social workers need to take a child-centred approach which also involves the family. While roles vary, core social work activities usually involve assessing needs and risks, advocating, counselling, strengthening families' resources and support networks and intervening in crisis situations. Social workers perform these duties in diverse settings, like in the community, as well as in schools, hospitals and government agencies. The MFT projects described in this section have been developed in different social services settings and tend to target families where children are at risk, have suffered or are suffering emotional and/or physical neglect and abuse. Some of the projects described in this chapter have also been developed and placed in child and adolescent mental health settings.

1. Early days

Overview

This eight-session MFT project (Morris, 2017) takes place at weekly intervals, with each session lasting 2 hours, facilitated by two practitioners. The project is for parents who have experienced anxiety, depression or other such difficulties following the birth of their child which are felt to be impacting their parenting. They may struggle with specific issues related to their infants or babies (newborn to 12 months), including sleep disturbances, feeding problems, difficulty settling and so on. Engagement often involves a home visit to explain about the group and answer any questions. If appropriate, the health visitor or other trusted professional can join. The focus of the work is to reduce the stigma new parents with mental health issues often experience and to promote the parents' capacity to mentalize their child and themselves. This sometimes involves linking current difficulties with past experiences of being parented. The room is set up with the chairs pushed to the sides and several large, clean, colourful baby mats placed on the floor in the

DOI: 10.4324/9781003442424-9

centre of the room. A few simple baby toys such as rattles as well as soft toys are scattered on the floor. There is a table with water, tea and coffee and warm water to heat bottles. Wet wipes and tissue as well as cushions to support breast feeding are also available in the room. As parents arrive in the room, they remove their shoes and sit on the floor. Whilst breast or bottle feeding, they can sit on a chair if they prefer. It is generally mothers and infants who attend this group, with the possibility of scheduling additional sessions when partners are invited. Interpreters and extended family members, for example, maternal grandmothers, are often also present. The group follows the same structure each week, with time allocated and themes selected differently according to the group's self-defined priorities.

1. **Settling in** – about 10 mins. Parents make their babies feel comfortable. Food is ordered.
2. **Singing a welcome song to the babies** – about 10 mins. This serves many functions, including to signal the beginning of the session, to welcome each infant as a being in their own right, to facilitate differentiation between carer and infant and to disinhibit parents and build their confidence. Welcoming songs include singing 'hello' as a group to each baby in turn, for example, '*Hello Zara, hello Zara, hello Zara, it's nice to see you here!*'
3. **'Catch-up' on week** – about 20 mins. This an opportunity for parents to share experiences and to talk to each other about specific challenges, as well as progressing towards more general goals, such as using the support of the extended family or enjoying time with their child. Whilst their discussions take place, the practitioners may draw attention to specific interactions between parents and infants, as well as making links, if appropriate, between the past and present issues in the parents' lives and highlighting positive coping strategies.
4. **MFT activity** – around 30 mins. This part of the group is more structured, with specific therapeutic aims, above all improving their capacity to mentalize their baby. The activities also help parents to move away from a position of being preoccupied with their own internal experiences. Following are a few examples of suitable activities.

Baby speed dating

The parents are asked to form an inner and outer circle, with their babies on their laps, and are invited to talk on a topic for a defined period of time before moving one seat so that they sit opposite another parent. However, rather than interviewing one another, the parents interview each other's babies, with the parent speaking on behalf of the baby: '*We would like you to interview the baby in front of you about their particular likes and dislikes for 2 minutes*'. The mother of the 'interviewed' baby has to answer the question on behalf of the baby. The pair swap roles before rotating and being asked to address the same question. The duration of this task can be shortened with each 'round', from 2 minutes to 1 minute, then again for 30 seconds and last for 10 seconds. This tends to create a lot of energy and laughter.

This activity helps parents to practice mentalizing skills, including differentiation, as it is made explicit that the baby's likes and dislikes are quite different from the carers.

Lucky dip

When introducing this activity, the practitioners state that they have written a range of different statements on separate pieces of paper. These are placed in a box with a hole in the lid. The babies are asked to take a paper from the lucky dip box, with the assistance of their parent, and read it to the parent next to them, who is allowed to say *'pass'* if they do not want to answer the questions and issues implied in the statement. The questions either pertain to the parents' transitions to motherhood (*'before I had a baby I spent most of my day . . . '; 'the biggest thing that has changed in my life since having a baby is . . . ') and the problems that have led to them coming to the group (for example, 'I first realized that I was having difficulties when . . . '; 'my biggest hope in attending this group is that . . . ').* There can also be less loaded and more neutral statements to which parents are meant to respond, for example, around likes and dislikes. The activity encourages group cohesion and the sharing of experiences in a non-threatening manner.

Baby as a film director

The parents are asked to design a storyboard for a film about their baby's life from the child's perspective. The film should begin in utero and finish with the child as an adult. The story boards are then shared with the group. Group discussion can focus on what needs to happen in the short and long term to help the child realize these dreams. The exercise can also provoke discussion over how much influence a parent has over a child's future.

Keep it in or throw it out

This activity promotes agency and reflection. Parents write on Post-It Notes three things about the way that they were parented that they would like to pass onto their child and three things that they would not. They then share these with the group. They take the Post-Its detailing the parenting practices they would like to 'keep' home with them, and, if they choose, they can throw the ones they would like to leave behind into a box in the middle of the room or leave them in the room after they leave.

Baby massage/stimulation

An instructional video on baby massage is watched, and various sensory toys, such as light- and sound-making toys and feathers, are brought into the room. Parents are instructed to interact with their babies using light, sound and touch and report back to the group what their baby liked and what they didn't. The practitioners make video recordings of some interactions for later viewing and reflection.

Mind scans

A session for both parents. The birth parents and their partners are divided into separate groups. Each group completes the activity (see Chapter 6) for their partner. Each set of parents then presents to the whole group their mind scans, and their partner reflects on what is accurate and what is less accurate. The discuss what have they learnt and what will they do with the new knowledge.

5. **Reflections** – around 10 minutes. The practitioners engage in a conversation in front of the families, reflecting on the work, bringing their different perspectives and making links, which the group members respond to if they wish. Video recordings of the groups as they work and parent–infant interactions are often reviewed and integrated into the reflections section (this section often needs to be extended slightly when video feedback is used).
6. **Singing a farewell song to the babies** – about 5 minutes. This signals the end of the session and builds on the benefits outlined previously.
7. **Parents and babies have lunch.** This part of the programme takes place without the practitioners being present, and it allows parents to build relationships and use mutual support in a less formal way. Different types of conversations evolve in the absence of professionals, and, as the group progresses, parents often exchange contact details to form social relationships and/or friendships outside the group context.

2. Kidstime – MFT with young carers and their families

Another application of MFT, implemented in both social services and health care settings are the Mental Health Matters Workshops, later re-named Kidstime Workshops, developed by Cooklin (2006) and his colleagues (Bishop et al., 2002) and now also known as Our Time. These projects are designed as a social intervention for dependent children of mentally ill parents and their families, with very specific goals (see Box 9).

Box 9   The goals of Kidstime workshops

- To help children and young people gain understandable explanations of their parents' mental illness and the behaviour in the parent which may be associated with this – whilst taking account of the child's own knowledge about the parent's condition

- To help children to gain more understanding and knowledge about mental illness and its treatment
- To provide an opportunity for children to address their fears, such as that they might 'catch' the illness, that they 'caused' the illness, that the parents may die from the illness and/or that they will not see their parent again
- To diminish the children's social isolation: learning that they are not 'the only ones' with the problem, meeting other young people with similar experiences
- To help the parents who suffer from mental illness to find a medium within which the illness and its impact can be discussed between themselves and their children
- To rebalance the children's 'inverted' role as carers within the family
- To share the load of responsibility with one or more adults
- To provide opportunities to engage in pleasurable age-appropriate activities with other young people
- To help the parents to access or rediscover their pride, confidence and competencies as parents
- To help the children experience their parents responding in a more positive manner

A major aim of the approach is to help children improve their resilience and their ability to protect their own mental health. Resilience studies have shown that children adapt better to a range of stressful situations if they feel less isolated and if they can develop a mental picture of the source of their anxiety or distress. However, many parents with mental illness attempt to protect their children from discussing their illness, and the Kidstime workshops explicitly challenge that stance: parents are supported to discuss mental health issues with their children, who learn about mental illness through discussion, drama and games, as well as exploring myths and fears about parental mental illness and combating stigma (Cooklin et al., 2011). The workshops enable children to be 'just children' and not to take on any adult responsibilities.

In their once-monthly meetings, the workshops incorporate several elements: they bring children and parents *together* around the topic of mental illness rather than professionals engaging with them separately, as so often tends to be the case. In the joined-up Kidstime setting, the mutual influences of parental mental illness on children and children's responses on parents can begin to be discussed and addressed. The intervention is not designated as a 'therapy', to avoid children feeling that they are in need of therapy. By contrast, the term 'workshop' suggests a relaxed and non-judgemental space for families to come together to learn and talk about mental illness, without fears about shame, guilt or stigma. A major aim is to diminish the social isolation which children of parents with mental illness often experience.

Format and structure

The workshops consist of monthly 2½ hour meetings for up to 15 families. Creative activities, drama and discussion are employed to address children's lack of knowledge and confusion about mental health problems and to encourage communication between parents and children. The workshops also provide a space for parents to socialize and support each other. Each workshop has a theme, such as 'diagnosis', 'treatment', 'voices groups' or 'young carers'. At least two practitioners are required to facilitate the workshops, and more depending on the size of the group and the ages of the children. If children younger than 3 years are present, then at least 2 practitioners need to facilitate the children's group. An example of a possible timetable for a Kidstime workshop is presented in Box 10.

Box 10   Timetable of Kidstime workshop

17.00 Families arrive – informal encounters
17.15 Icebreaker activity
17.30 Parallel parents' and children's group
18.30 Pizza eating
18.50 Viewing of children's work by parents
19.15 Joint reflections
19.30 End

After an icebreaker activity, children and parents are initially separated. The parents participate in a discussion group, talking to each other about various themes, like their illness and its effects, including those on their children. They share experiences and discuss their role as parents rather than being patients. While the parents are engaged in conversation, the children, with the help of a practitioner, make a little film or write sketches which have specific themes, such as 'living with the illness', 'when help is not helpful', 'when nobody listens' or 'fear'. They can also do paintings, collages or other forms of art that express their preoccupations. About 60 to 90 minutes need to be allowed for children to complete these activities, and this will also have to include rehearsal time, as the work of the children is then displayed to the parents. Towards the last part of the workshop, everyone gathers for eating pizza, which is a popular highlight for children and parents alike. The sketches are then performed in front of the parents, or, if a little film or other pieces of art have been made, these are shown to them. This is followed by a general discussion exploring the various themes and connecting them to the parents' group, which has gone on in parallel to the children's group. Sometimes families make overt links with issues portrayed in the play or film and the reality at home. At other times, it is just left for everyone to draw their own conclusions.

3. MFT for adoptive families

Overview and format

This project has been devised for adoptive families with children aged 5–11 who have suffered early relational trauma. Relational trauma can have a significant impact on their attachment representations and capacity to mentalize, including attention control, emotional regulation and trusting others. Adoptive parents can experience their children as controlling, unpredictable and/or disconnected, and this can place a significant strain on family relationships. They can often feel overwhelmed, hopeless and judged as a result of their children's behaviour. Adoptive children can similarly feel unsafe, misunderstood and stigmatized. This project brings families together so that they can share their experiences, build social support and engage in activities that promote mentalization, family relationships and identity. Much of the work with the children happens at an implicit level, whereas there is the possibility of moving to a more reflective level with parents. For this reason, some of the groups provide separate spaces for parents and children. The group is run in the evenings in a community setting. It starts with a 1 × 2-hour 'taster session'. Families who wish to continue then attend 7 × 2-hour fortnightly groups. They are welcome to attend with extended family or other closely involved members of their support network. Each group begins with 15 minutes unstructured 'snack time'. The group then meets for a brief activity all together. Depending on the session, the group then stays together or separates into parents and children's groups, always coming together for a 10-minute group activity at the end before going home. The process of parents and children separating and reuniting is used explicitly and implicitly as a therapeutic tool. Photographs are taken over the course of each group and used to stimulate mentalizing throughout and produce a gallery at the end.

Session overview

Session 1: 'Taster session'

Icebreaker: Finding Your Place. The families are invited to line up in order of height without talking.

Activity: Posters: '*We would like you to make a poster to advertise this group. Imagine if this was the best-ever, most helpful group you had ever been to; what would the poster say?'* Parents and children are separated into different rooms. After 40 minutes the parents and children are reunited and present their posters to one another. It is made clear that if a child needs a parent at any point during the group, then the parent goes to the child group rather than the child joining the parent group. This allows parents the space to relax a little and speak freely.

Ending game: The final 10 minutes of the group finishes with the *Who Has Ever . . . ?* activity.

Task: The families are encouraged to have a conversation on the way home about what they liked and didn't like about the group and whether they would like to come back.

Session 2: Feelings fish

Welcome back and rule-making: Each family is given 10 minutes to decide four rules that they would like the group to work by and then invited to share with the rest of the group, who decide which ones they would like to keep.

Activity: Feelings Fish. The practitioners are also given a chance to work on an individual family level during this activity. After 20 minutes, the group is encouraged to get up and move around to find another group member from a different family to find out about each other's fish. This is repeated one more time before the practitioner carefully collects up the fish, explaining that we will come back to them next time.

Ending game: Musical Statues.

Task: Notice when each other feel like their fish at home.

Session 3: Smoke signals

Icebreaker: Smoke Signals

Activity: Seascape: a big picture on the wall with brightly coloured coral, a dangerous whirlpool, big open sea, long dense reeds, caves to hide in and so on. The group are invited to work in pairs (one adult and one child) to find out where each others' feelings fish (from previous week) likes to live and why: are they happy there, or would they prefer to live somewhere else? How would they get there? Children should choose an adult who is not their parent, who then presents about the fish to the rest of the group.

Ending game: Shark Attack! The children sit with their legs out straight under an opened parachute (or large blanket, with shoes removed). The children are asked who would like to be a 'shark'. They go under the parachute in the middle and have to 'attack' by pulling someone's toes. The parents are asked to nominate two 'lifeguards'. Their job is to patrol the perimeter and anticipate the shark attack, rescuing the person before they are pulled under. The rest of the parents watch, trying to alert the lifeguard when they see a potential attack. Children are told if you would not like to get caught you can choose to sit with your legs crossed.

Task: At home, talk about what it felt like to be save/be saved/attack.

Session 4: Time apart

Icebreaker: Wink Murder.

Parents' group: The adults are bought together to think about their experiences in the group so far, encouraged to mentalize themselves and their children and to think about how to transfer their understanding to the home setting. Video recordings can be used.

Children's group – Talent Show: Children are told they will have time next week to finish rehearsals before the actual performance. This activity promotes children's sense of self and agency. It celebrates their strengths, and it allows the focus to be on something other than the fact that they are adopted.

Ending game: The group is invited to choose any of the games we have played so far or to make one of their own.

Task: Goals set in the parents' group.

Session 5: The X factor

The same format as session 4. The parents are encouraged to 'report back' to the group on the changes they have made and to decide on things to try over the next 2 weeks. The parents start a 'support notice board' (flip chart paper) where they share details of support agencies and resources that they have found helpful. This is brought to all subsequent sessions for parents to add to, and all parents are invited to take a photo of the flip chart on their phone at the last session. The group finishes with the children performing their talent show. They are all given the same amount of time, and each child's performance is cheered by the whole group.

Task: Plan together how the child can show off their talents more often.

Session 6: Stranded on an island!

Icebreaker: Duck, Duck, Goose!

Activity: Family Rucksack. In this variation of the activity, all group members are given an A3 photocopy of an empty rucksack. It is explained that the children will be asked to draw pictures in the bag of the five most important things that their parents would bring if they were told they were going to be stranded on a desert island for a month. The parents are told that they should do the same for their children. Again, they will be working in separate rooms.

Ending game: The group is invited to choose any of the games we have played so far to finish or to invent a new one.

Task: Talk as a family about trips you have taken, now or in the past, and trips you would like to take in the future.

Session 7: Animal families

Activity: Animal Families. Time is taken over this activity at every stage, where themes of belonging and difference in families are particularly pertinent. The families then plan for the final session.

Ending game: The group is invited to choose any of the games we have played so far to finish or invent a new one.

Task: Find some pictures of your family when you are at your happiest and talk about these memories. How can you make more memories like this?

Session 8: Goodbye celebration

Popping Balloons activity (for those who don't like a bang, the air can be let out slowly). The families then proceed with the ending session celebration in the way they planned. At some point the practitioners show a slideshow 'photo gallery' displaying the families' journey along all the sessions. This promotes integration and coherent narrative as families remember their time together.

4. Family day units and intensive specialized multi-family therapy

Family day units are a particularly intensive form of MFT, as families attend for whole days over months. They are engaged as experts in what could also be termed a 'collaborative family programme' (Fraenkel, 2006). The first day unit for families, a publicly funded mental health project, was pioneered in the 1980s at the Marlborough Family Service in London (Asen et al., 1982) and inspired in part by the structural approach (Minuchin, 1974). It has served as a model for similar projects which have been developed in several countries, some of which are based in mental health services, with others located in social services settings. Family day units have proved to be helpful for the work with 'multi-problem families', a label employed to describe multiply disadvantaged and marginalized families with severe relationship problems. Social isolation, poor education, alcohol and substance misuse, intra-family violence and severe psychiatric disorders in more than one generation are all usually present at the same time. The children of these multiply disadvantaged families tend to come to the attention of social services, education welfare and child and adolescent mental health services, with the latter often avoiding providing input because the families are seen as 'treatment-resistant' if not 'impossible'. Not infrequently family courts are involved and require the assessment of parenting capacity. Family day units are excellent facilities to undertake comprehensive assessments, commissioned by social services and/or by court, as the intensity and duration of their stay permit close observation of family dynamics and parenting capacity.

Putting between six and eight of these families together under one roof, for whole days over a period of several months, in a day unit for families, a kind of 'therapeutic community of dysfunctional families' (Cooklin et al., 1983), seemed a way forward all those years ago. The very structured daily timetable aims to counteract the often seemingly chaotic ways multi-problem families live their daily lives. The many quick context changes throughout the day, from being members of a large group setting to taking part in single-family work, from participating in small buzz-groups to having to attend a fathers-only group, from speed-dating to becoming members of a reflecting team – all this requires families and their members to adopt different positions and roles in the space of only a few hours. This activates many parents to take better responsibility to manage the mundane tasks of daily living – like preparing meals, getting their children to eat, clearing up afterwards and always keeping an eye on their children. The structure of the programme reflects this by deliberately making the management of ordinary family life a major focus of the work. A typical timetable of a day in a family day unit is described in Box 11.

Box 11　Family day unit timetable

9.00　Families arrive
9.15　*Speed Dating*
9.40　Planning meeting and selection of activity
10.00　MFT activity (e.g., *Family Clay Sculpts, Family Life River*)
11.00　Break
11.15　Parallel parents' and children's group (e.g., discussing impact of ill-ness/alcohol on family, managing anger and frustration, creating appropriate boundaries, etc.)
12.00　Preparation of lunch, eating and clearing up
13.30　Icebreaker (e.g., *Amoeba Game, Tug of War*)
13.45　Group activity (e.g., *How Others See You, Labelling Oneself, Feelings Fish*)
15.00　Reflections meeting
15.30　Finish

Whole-day MFT, with its inbuilt frequent transitions from one working context and activity to the next, is quite a challenge – not only for families but also for staff! When families arrive in a day unit each morning, the children need to be settled by the parents, and this allows the observation of their ability to prioritize their children's needs above their own. With children placed in local authority care, it is their foster carers who bring them to the day unit and hand them over to their parents. This can evoke rather poignant encounters between parents and foster carers, sometimes with the children being directly exposed to such conflicts, and, if so, this will be addressed then and there by the practitioners by encouraging the adults to mentalize their children and themselves. In the planning meeting at the beginning of the day, each family is asked to discuss and plan how they are going to use the day to address the issues that they want to work on. Those families who state that they are the 'innocent victims' of misguided social workers will be asked to address those issues which the children's social workers have identified. A plan for the day is then co-constructed by families and practitioners, often around specific themes such as 'being excluded', 'dominating everything', 'not trusting anybody', 'nobody ever listens' or 'feeling alone and misunderstood'.

Once a particular theme for the day has been chosen and agreed upon, an MFT activity will be chosen, usually by the practitioners. This can consist of playing a board game, making a family picture or collage, carrying out homework set by the school or choosing some other suitable activity as described in Chapter 6. All these activities require the family members to work together and for someone to lead the activity or play and to ensure that turn taking takes place. During this time, the practitioners are in the 'eagle position' and may approach a family briefly to share an observation or make a suggestion, only to withdraw again and leave the family to itself. In a subsequent reflective round, families tell each other what they have done and also what they may have observed, not only about their own interactions but also those in other families. Often a theme emerges which can then be explored in a subsequent multi-family activity. Typical themes are: 'being excluded', 'dominating everything', 'nobody is in charge', 'nobody ever listens' and 'enjoying being together'. When the experimental phase of the activity is over, families are encouraged in small sub-groups to reflect on what they have experienced and perhaps even earned. This is followed by a short break, requiring parents to take care of their children, who, by this stage, are often quite excited and possibly dysregulated, requiring their parents to take control. After the break, parallel parents' and children's groups can be formed, with the adults discussing issues related to the theme of the day. The children are often given creative tasks that also relate to the same theme.

Families bring their own food, and around noon each family begins to prepare their own lunch. The actual preparation and cooking of food whilst having to involve or supervise children can be taxing for parents and replicate difficult domestic situations. Parents – and often their children – are also responsible for washing and clearing up afterwards, triggering potentially fraught interactions between members of different families when sharing kitchen utensils or arguing whose job it is to clear up a specific 'mess'. During the afternoon there is the opportunity for other activities, usually involving all families together. It is also possible to go on an outing with all the families, be that to a local park or shopping centre, enabling practitioners to observe how parents manage their, at times very challenging, children in public. Here typical problematic family scenarios are spontaneously enacted, and, if these are filmed, they can be viewed and reflected upon later in a video feedback session later that day. At the end of each day there is a brief reflective round, when experiences and observations are shared and goals for the next few days set, including how to transfer the 'lessons' learnt to each family's own home.

Families often attend day units for 4–6 months, and occasionally longer. Interestingly, many families who state at the outset that they had been 'forced' to attend find it difficult to leave when their time is up. They report that this intensive experience has helped them to overcome their social isolation and enabled them to make new friendships. Many also report that the experience of being helpful to other parents and children has made them become aware that they have resources that might be difficult to employ within one's own family but can be of good use to others.

Intensive specialized multi-family therapy (ISMFT) is a related way of intervening with multi-problem families, and the approach can be described as a 'last resort' before decisions about the removal of children from their parents' care are considered (Overbeek et al., 2023). It is an integrated therapy for multi-problem families which is based on the Family Day Unit approach described previously, with added solution-focused interventions. ISMFT is a day treatment for 6 hours, taking place 3 days a week for 7 weeks. This adds up to 21 days for parents and 18 days for children. This form of intervention has been found to improve family functioning (van Beek et al., 2023).

5. Lighthouse parenting MFT

Overview

The Lighthouse Parenting Programme (Byrne et al., 2019) was developed to promote mentalizing modes of thinking and parenting in high-risk groups, specifically parents of children 'on the edge of care'. It aims to enhance parents' general capacity to mentalize and in particular to mentalize their children, to enhance attunement in parent–child relationship, to promote secure attachment and reduce disorganization and to reduce risk of harm and trans-generational transmission of psychopathology. The Lighthouse Parenting Programme (LPP) is a manualized, 20-week course for parents, combining group and individual sessions (Byrne et al., 2019; Volkert et al., 2022). The programme is suitable for families with children up to the age of 10. It was developed specifically for the parents of children on child in need or child protection plans or in family court proceedings, many of whom have experienced early developmental and/or subsequent traumas, often within the context of disorganized attachment relationships. The LPP addresses the complexity of establishing meaningful engagement with parents who understandably lack trust in others and in agencies and institutions. It is informed by trauma and attachment research and adopts a mentalizing approach to intervention to help parents achieve a better balance in their management and regulation of their own feelings and thoughts and support them to see their child more clearly. The core metaphor is that of the parent as a 'lighthouse' whose light of attention can bathe a child in the warmth of their curiosity and reliably 'find' the child's mind to respond sensitively to their needs, bringing the child consistently into 'safe harbour' as often as is needed (held in mind). The strong visual metaphors help parents and children grasp key insights on their relationship with the child and on factors informing their parenting.

The LPP helps parents approach their child with a curious, wanting-to-know mentalizing stance, the 'illuminating beam'. This helps them to recognize where their own mentalizing as a parent can fail and when too much certainty about their child's inner world – which can be prone to distortion – replaces curiosity, a phenomenon which can be described as the 'projecting beam'. The LPP gives parents skills to recognize such moments and, when they happen, to attempt to restore their own mentalizing capacity to gain clearer sight of the child.

Format and structure

Lighthouse Parenting MFT (LP-MFT) is an adaptation of the original programme by including children in some of the sessions. It is a semi-manualized intervention consisting of 12 sessions, of which 8 are parents only and 4 whole families. Two parent-only groups which explore specific themes and how these may be relevant for parenting their child are followed by a multi-family group which involves the children, allowing the parents to put their 'learning' into practice. This process is repeated three times over the course of the group. The parents only sessions last 2 hours, whereas the multi-family events last 3 hours. Sessions take place in fortnightly intervals. They each have a specific focus, with themes and content for the 'parents only' meetings.

Session overview

Session 1: Parents only: Introduction to the model and overview
Session 2: Parents only: The concept of the 'safe harbour' and how parents can create one for their child

The first two sessions introduce key concepts of the lighthouse programme, including the parent as lighthouse that holds the child in mind via illuminating and scanning beams. The 'not-knowing stance' and the 'wanting to know stances' are explained and explored, with the emphasis on vigilance and safeguarding. Weak and absent beams and their sequelae are also discussed.

Session 3: Parents and children: Exploring the lighthouse metaphors

Families meet each other via an icebreaker exercise, followed by *Speed Dating*. The parents then present the colourful lighthouse images to the children and get their ideas and associations about each image. The parents use the images to explain to their child the idea of a safe harbour (base). Each parent makes a lighthouse armband with their child and puts it on to symbolize that they are their child's lighthouse. Stories about lighthouses, rough seas and safe harbours are told and briefly enacted. Parents explain what they think and feel when a boat that carries the children is out of sight. They speculate what the children might think and feel if they can no longer see their parents. A storm on the sea is role played, and parents and children mentalize themselves and each other, focusing on how they can get help and what they need to feel safe. Towards the end, both children and parents consider whom they want to recruit to their 'crew' for intersession work, and together they consider composing a sea journal to document their experience and what they have learnt, which they can continue to complete at home, for example, each night before going to bed. Key themes and interactions are 'bookmarked' for later reflection. Video recordings can be made for later reflection.

Session 4: Parents: Reflections about the previous MFT session, speculating about children's feelings and needs
Session 5: Parents only: Being confused and other forms of non-mentalizing
Session 6: Parents and children: Leaving and returning to the safe harbour

In role plays, preparations are made on what to take on the journey, like packing a survival rucksack for all eventualities, deciding what is important to whom and why. This requires that the parents and children mentalize each other. This is followed by the families building together an (imaginary) boat for the journey, using a few props. Roles are allocated for all those 'on board'. The journey starts, and safety measures are discussed, with a focus on the potential fears of both parents and children. The families decide on the course of the journey and which challenges are encountered: rough seas, sea monsters, strange new lands. They work together to manage these challenges, eventually returning, safe and sound, back to harbour. Key moments and interactions are 'bookmarked', and recordings can also be made for reflection at the next parents' group. The parents and children are then separated for a brief time, primarily for the parents to reflect together. The families then come together to talk about their day. The practitioners may facilitate this discussion by thinking of key questions and making a playful context for them to be asked. At the end of the group, the families report back from their respective sea journals and consider what adventures lie ahead in the forthcoming weeks.

Session 7: Parents only: Reflections about the previous MFT session, memories and needs
Session 8: Parents only: Feeling lost and not wanting to be found
Session 9 Parents and children: Drifting on a raft

The group begins with the *Smoke Signals* activity. Parents then explain to children what a raft is, and each family builds their own raft and thinks of a story, preferably informed by personal experiences. In separate children's and parents' groups, the thoughts and feelings evoked by the activity are discussed and then shared together in the big group. Practitioners ensure that the parents listen to and respond to what the children voice. Parents then 'cross-foster' other children and complete the *Feelings Fish* activity and present their work to the whole group.

Finally, the group shares entries from their sea journals. Key themes and interactions are 'bookmarked' for later reflection and video recordings are also made for later reflection. The transfer task is for each child to pretend to be on a raft on one day between sessions; the parents have to guess when that is and respond to the child's needs and document this.

*Session 10: Parents only: Reflections about the previous MFT session, managing
    internal and external conflicts*
Session 11: Parents: Becoming perturbed and confused
Session 12: Parents and children: Developing trust

Parents and children role play what happens when their ship hits a fog bank. Families then discuss what can be done when one is confused. Who can lead one when there is no light? This is followed by the *Blind Trust* activity. After reflecting about their respective experiences, a parents' and a children's group are set up. The parents talk about their experiences of their children not trusting them – and the other way round. They discuss strategies of generating trust. Each child in their group draws a trust pyramid, placing those they trust most at the bottom and those they trust least at the top of the pyramid. When the activity is finished, they are cross-fostered and show and explain their trust pyramid to the 'foster parent'. The group finishes with a ritual with all the lighthouse armbands, *Feelings Fish* and sea journals being displayed and each person saying something about the items in turn and what they have enjoyed most about their journey.

6. Addressing high-conflict parenting

Overview

Chronic and unresolved inter-parental conflict can negatively impact children's wellbeing, and several single-family and multi-family projects have been developed over the past decade for these children and their separated parents. Parental separation itself does not necessarily harm children, but repeated and long-term exposure of children can amount to severe emotional abuse and neglect, placing them at risk of developing mental illness and being susceptible to masking and not being able to sustain trusting relationships in the future (Asen & Morris, 2020). Children in these scenarios literally remain caught in the middle between the warring parents, and they can feel so conflicted and confused by each parent's demonizing narrative of the other that they will 'pick a side', forming a strong alliance with one parent and becoming increasingly reluctant to spend time with the other.

The No Kids in the Middle MFT programme

No Kids in the Middle (NKM) is a semi-structured multi-family programme that aims to help separated parents experiencing high conflict move away from their polarized disputes to find new ways of communicating that place their child's welfare at the centre (Van Lawick & Visser, 2015; Visser & Van Lawick, 2021). It can be offered as a stand-alone intervention, as a pre-cursor or as a follow-up to individual family work, depending on the needs of the family. The intervention is designed for children aged 4–12, though for practical reasons it is sometimes necessary for older or younger siblings to attend as well.

Structure of the NKM programme

Families are seen for two 'intake' sessions prior to the group, where they are given information about the programme and a 'taste' of what the group involves. The family is assessed for eligibility, and they also decide whether the programme is right for them. Approximately six families work together in an MFT format over eight weekly sessions; each session lasts 2 hours. Parents and children work in parallel in two separate groups in the same building, coming together for a short break halfway through each session. Two practitioners facilitate each of the two groups.

Work with parents

The approach centres around key principles:

- keeping the child in mind at all times;
- the involvement of the families' social networks;
- 'letting go' and acceptance (for example, by parents accepting that they are unable to control the other parent);
- recognizing destructive patterns of communication and their impact;
- recognizing and managing trauma, grief and stress;
- tolerating ambivalence.

When the child's experience is lost from the parent's minds, it is the practitioners' role to gently bring the child back into focus. Towards this aim, the child is represented by a small chair at the centre of the room throughout the parents' group. Participation in the group involves the parents engaging with group activities aimed at eliciting feelings and perspectives and safely experimenting with new interactions and creative presentations. For high-conflict couples post-separation, therapeutic discussion can fail to enable parents to fully understand what it is like for their child to be caught in the 'crossfire' of conflict. While parents often 'already know' that conflict can harm their child, they are nevertheless so preoccupied with intense feelings towards their ex-partner that they cannot hold the child's experience in mind (Hertzmann et al., 2016). Given this, work at an experiential level can succeed where discussion has failed. Parents are given homework tasks at the end of each session, which they are usually asked to complete with the support of their social network.

The children's group

In the children's group, a key part of the approach is to maintain a sense of playfulness in children, and they are supported to talk, play and be creative around various relevant themes (e.g., 'divided loyalties' or 'having two homes'). At the beginning of the group, the children are introduced to the idea of working on a project, taking any form they like, on their own or together, that reflects something about their experience of being 'in the middle' (this can be, for example, a poem or artwork). They are offered the chance to share this with the parents' group, if they want to, at the end of the intervention, but there is no obligation. It is made clear to the children that it is the adults' responsibility to 'do the work'. Children may also draw support from one another.

The social network

One challenge when working with high-conflict parents is the need to 'bring on board' the families' social network. Unless this happens, changes parents make can be undermined by the wider support network, who can maintain polarized perspectives, refuse to forgive transgressions and perpetuate unhelpful patterns of communication (Visser et al., 2017). It is a key part of the NKM model that the parents' social network (new partners, family, friends) is included at the outset of the intervention.

To this end, there is a Social Network Meeting at the beginning of the programme where each parent can invite two to five people. The network is invited again halfway through the programme, this time without the parents, to discuss progress and share experiences.

Overview of the programme

Social network meeting: Both parents attend with the social network. The children do *not* attend

Group 1: Parents' topic: Loving patterns and destructive patterns

Children's topic: Introduction to the group

Group 2: Parents' topic: Children in the centre, parents role play being the child caught in the midst of conflict

Children's topic: How it was in the past, how it is now and how you would like it to be

Group 3: Parents' topic: Parents jointly write a non-demonizing story of their separation to share with their children

Children's topic: Conflict: what does it mean to you, and what does it look like in your life?

Group 4: Parents' topic: New solutions for old problems. Each parent brings a current co-parenting problem which the other parents help them to solve

Children's topic: Divided loyalties

Group 5: Parents' topic: New solutions for old problems continued

Children's topic: Planning/rehearsing for presentations

Interim social network meeting: The same network that attended the initial network meeting attend without the parents to review progress

Group 6: Children's presentation of their work to parents and/or a message to their parents about what they have done/felt during the group

Group 7: Parents' presentations: a message to the children about what they have learned in the group

Group 8: Goodbye party

Chapter 10

MFT projects in schools

Overview

The use of multi-family groups in schools is intended to help children and young people who are having difficulties with learning because their emotional and/or behavioural challenges distract them from the core teaching and learning required to be a successful student (Dawson & McHugh, 1994; Asen et al., 2001). Common features are the children's difficulties in their interactions with other students and finding the classroom and playground relationships particularly problematic, where they can become quickly dysregulated and angry and then increasingly isolated, with few or no friends. School staff find themselves in difficult positions with these students, feeling the need to supervise them at all times in order to minimize the disruptive impact on the other children and to keep them and others safe. This can typically result in the students having qualified adults assigned to them, like teaching assistants, frequently not only for some or all the lessons but also and during break and playtimes. It can also result in students spending significant amounts of time away from the classroom, for example, in 'inclusion' rooms. However, the act of providing such intense monitoring and support can isolate the child from their peers even more, making them appear and feel even more different. This impacts further their ability to engage in the classroom and can remove the opportunity to develop the relational skills necessary for independence and autonomy. Difficulties with the student's behaviour and/or integration at school can place significant stress on parent–school communications and relationships, with parents often feeling blamed, misunderstood or unsupported by schools. Schools, on the other hand, become frustrated at what they can see as a lack of engagement or co-operation of the parent. The child/student can experience contradictory or confusing messages about any problematic situation, which can lead to further dysregulation.

School-based MFT is designed to help overcome the need for children to be dependent on the support and supervision of an adult throughout the day and the need for exclusion/time out. School-based MFT does not require children or their families to have a diagnosis and hopefully avoids medicalizing them. Parents join multi-family work in schools primarily because they want to help their children change so that their engagement with learning and school improves. A major

DOI: 10.4324/9781003442424-10

consequence of participating in a school-based multi-family group is that often relationships and behaviours improve at home as well, even though this is at the outset not usually the key focus of the work. The approach also aims to develop mutual respect and collaboration across parent–teacher relationships in support of good outcomes for students.

MFT has been expanded to support different levels of need, for example, for students who are finding it difficult to engage in learning as a result of anxiety and low mood, in addition to behavioural and relational difficulties. Since the COVID epidemic, there has been a significant increase in children not attending school. For example, in 2021/22, 22.5% of pupils in the UK were recorded as 'persistently absent'. Often additional needs, including neurodiversity, are a significant contributory factor, impacting a student's ability to engage in school, for example, because of sensory overwhelm and the challenge of navigating social relationships in a neurotypical environment. Neurodivergent children are often targeted and bullied as well feeling the need to mask their difficulties, impacting their long-term emotional development. Social disadvantage, family stress (including parental conflict, parental mental health difficulties and parental substance abuse) and cultural factors (including experience of discrimination as a result of being in a minoritized group) also contribute significantly towards a child's ability to engage with school and learning.

In recent years there has been a lot more thought given to the need for schools to be trauma-informed environments (Thomas et al., 2019). Children who have experienced early relational trauma have been found to process information differently to those who have experienced 'good enough' parenting. Their brains have developed in in response to abusive and/or neglectful experiences: in order to keep safe, they tend to be hypervigilant to threat; they are not used to positive behaviour being rewarded, and so they have learned not to anticipate rewards; they are preoccupied with not making mistakes and so have impaired executive functioning; they work hard to avoid negative affect and so can have poor emotional regulation skills; and they often don't remember and integrate positive experiences to make a coherent narrative (McCrory & Viding, 2015). Whilst such strategies may well have been adaptive for some of these children in their early years, they can result in significant social and educational challenges in a mainstream school environment and low epistemic trust. So, while diagnosis per se does not organize MFT groups in school, practitioners work carefully to ensure that each child's individual difficulties and needs are 'seen' and understood (mentalized) in the multi-family setting and also in schools where MFT is implemented.

Over the last 40 years a whole spectrum of multifamily interventions in educational or school settings have been developed to meet the needs of students and their families. These can be grouped according to the intensity of the intervention: a low-intensity intervention is a family class which happens once a week for 2 to 3 hours. Medium-intensity family classes take place two to three mornings per week for 2 to 3 hours. A high-intensity family class tends to be part of a specialized mental health or educational facility, taking place four to five mornings per week for up to 3 hours. Finally, the most high-intensity intervention is the family school, which takes place five days a week, from 9 a.m. to 3 p.m. Family class and family school projects are not organized by diagnoses, but they require that each child's individual barriers to learning be mentalized and addressed, including barriers that are associated with a neurodevelopmental diagnosis and social, cultural and environmental factors.

1. The family class

The family class concept was developed many years ago in London (Dawson & McHugh, 1994; Asen et al., 2001), and it has since been implemented in many European countries and elsewhere. Typically, between six and eight children or young people and their families are selected to take part in a family class together with a teacher or other member of the school staff and a MFT practitioner. Involving a member of school staff further facilitates collaboration between parents and the school in the way they understand and support the children. It also brings with it the benefit of integrating principles of MFT and mentalizing across the broader school context. A family class usually lasts for a school term in the first instance, taking place once weekly and lasting between 90 minutes and 2, 3 or 5 hours. It can be delivered during normal school hours or after school finishes in a room in a mainstream primary or secondary school (Dawson & McHugh, 1994). The head teacher, head of year or pastoral lead selects each term between six and eight challenging students from different years and classes of their respective school, asking them and their parents to attend a family class for 10 to 12 weeks. It is possible for students to have a second term in a family class.

The potential participants for the family class, often disruptive students who present with challenging behaviours, are recruited by the year heads or the head of the school, who approach the parents first, explaining the model and motivating the parents or other primary carers to commit themselves attending a family class for a term. Not infrequently the parents may be told that unless there is a major change of the student's conduct, they may be permanently excluded. Prior to attending the family class, the children, young people and at least one of their adult family members meet all together with the family class leaders, and behavioural, educational and emotional wellbeing targets are set for each student. The process of agreeing to these targets is the first step in supporting the parent–school relationship, as the targets are jointly agreed upon and monitored by the parent, student and school. The targets can range from specific changes in behaviour to improved educational achievements. Examples are:

- to complete and hand in the homework on time;
- to keep their hands and feet to themselves;
- to raise their arm first before answering a question;
- to speak respectfully to the lunchtime supervisor;
- to help the disabled child move from one classroom to another;
- to let the class teacher know when stress levels at home interfere with learning;
- to come into school and to morning lessons.

No more than three or four targets are set for a student, and these are marked by teachers and other school staff on a daily or weekly basis on a scale from 1 to 4, with 4 being the top score for consistently meeting the specific target. The parents are requested to check the scores each day or week and to clarify with the teacher(s) any trouble that the child might have had. In this way a daily feedback loop is established between family and school, and the child experiences them working collaboratively. The scores are discussed in each family class. Once a child consistently obtains satisfactory scores on one target, a new target can be set. The consistent improvement in a student's score on behavioural and educational targets is a clear indicator that change has taken place. Furthermore, when children begin to consistently receive positive marks, it becomes easier to change their negative reputation at school. Initially the targets are primarily focused on the student's behaviour at school, but most parents opt sooner rather than later for doing the same at home, and specific home targets get drawn up with child and parent, focusing, for example, on eating, bedtimes, use of mobile phone and games and so on. Children often cannot resist the temptation to set targets for their parents, like not shouting at them, to be home when the child returns from school, to read a bedtime story with the child or for the parent not to use a mobile phone for specific periods in the afternoon or evening.

Structure and organization of the family class reflect the combined education and therapeutic context, including the physical setup of the classroom, the curriculum, the timetable and the various activities carried out. It is a school situation, enriched by parental presence and involvement. During the family class, the behaviours that may be causing the usual difficulties in the classroom tend to evolve spontaneously in full view of the parents. This is why one of the ingredients of the family class programme is a formal lesson which a qualified teacher conducts, with the parents observing the interactions between students and teacher from the back of the classroom. One parent may notice that their offspring is getting very frustrated because they are unable to complete a task and behave in a rude way towards a teacher, kicking over his chair and walking away. The parents can be asked to mentalize the child and teacher and form hypotheses about how and why the interactions developed. A standard timetable of a family class is set out in Box 12.

Box 12   Family class timetable

9.00 Icebreaker activity
9.15 Review of students' school targets. The parents' targets may also be discussed
9.45 Break
10.00 Formal lesson, with parents observing
10.45 Parents reflect on their observations
11.00 MFT activity (see subsequently)
11.45 Reflection and evaluation of the school day, preview of coming week

---

Typical themes that come up in family classes relate to managing rules and boundaries, emotional regulation, bullying, marginalization and discrimination and the parents' own history of attending school. The most commonly used MFT activities reflect these themes. They are: *Who Has Ever?; Bully, Bullied, Bystander; Press Conference; Escalation Clock; Life River; Family Constitution, Mood Barometer; Popping Balloons; Wrong-Hand Writing*. Family classes work best when they function as a closed group for the term, but during the subsequent term some students will have left the family class, and new students can be added. 'Graduate' parents and children who have attended previous MFT groups can help with recruitment and engagement. With school-based multi-family groups, it is also important to establish from the beginning rules around confidentiality and respect, as, especially in primary school, parents are likely to see each other frequently outside of the group and to know people in common.

2. Family school projects

Several family school projects have been developed over the years in different parts of Europe, employing a multi-family approach in a part- or full-time school setting. The first such project started in the 1990s in London at the Marlborough Family Service. Funded jointly by the local Health and Education services, the project was named Family Education Centre (Asen et al., 2001); the use of the term 'family school' was not permitted at the time. The project started when it was noticed that the needs of a considerable number of students could not be met by attending family classes: they just seemed to need more. Furthermore, students permanently excluded from mainstream schools also required an educational facility. Therefore, the creation of a 'family school' seemed a further sensible development to bring parents into schools and get them to be partners in the educational progress of their children. Being present in school for significant periods of time enabled them to learn first-hand about their children in an educational context and to experience how family issues were at times being re-enacted in school (Dawson & McHugh, 1994). A major aim for students attending the Family Education Centre was to eventually re-integrate them into a mainstream school once improvements in their behavioural and emotional presentations had taken place. This meant that they *had* to be on the roll of a mainstream school, and if a student had been permanently excluded, the local education authority was required to identify a school which the student could attend in the future once the required changes have been made. The reason for insisting on there being an identified school was to prevent the Family Education Centre to become an 'end of the road' institution, collecting society's marginalized and unwanted students. Hence it was agreed that students would sooner rather than later attend in parallel their identified mainstream school, if only for 1 hour per week at the outset and, once their presentations were improving, for increasingly long spells. Between 1995 and 2013, the Family Education Centre could at any time accommodate 10 students between the ages of 5 and 14 and their carers.

In 2014 the Family Education Centre was transferred to the Anna Freud Centre and became initially known as the Family School (London), a unique alternative provision for up to 48 students, aged 5 to 14, who had been excluded from mainstream schools. To get the required accreditation of becoming a state-registered school, the model had to be adapted to allow for a full 5-day attendance of students over the period of one whole school year. Parents are not required to attend every day, but they do need to do so for a minimum of 1 full day per week. The family school aims to combine high-quality teaching and learning with a fully integrated mental health curriculum in a non-stigmatizing environment. Reintegration to mainstream school remains the major aim. Having families – and indeed students – for a whole day permits much observation of typical situations that occur in schools between teachers and students, between students and students, between parents and teachers – and more. The use of video recordings allows these situations to be viewed once the initial arousal has subsided and effective mentalizing has kicked in again.

Parental participation one day a week is mandatory. The children start the day by attending the respective classes. The parents meet at 9.30 am for a joint breakfast and have an informal discussion of what the week has been like for them and their children. At 10.00, parent learning starts, a bespoke programme, with a curriculum specifically designed together with parents, to attend to issues that are important to them and their children. It is run weekly, with a 20-week curriculum cycle, permitting newly joining parents to enter at different points throughout the school year. The aim is to help parents gain greater understanding of their own and their children's emotional worlds and related mental health issues, as well as covering various other topics that are important for family life. Another aim is to boost self-esteem of parents as they work through the material, as many of the parents attending the family school have themselves not succeeded at school. Parents are consulted on what they would like to learn about, and they co-construct the curriculum. Their top issue is about the scope and limitations of their children receiving a medical diagnosis and managing their difficult behaviours. The learning is then later that day translated into action via the various MFT activities. For example, following a formal presentation about different diagnoses and their scope and limitations, a lively debate often ensues about how diagnoses can affect children and other family members. There are usually mixed views as to whether a child receiving a diagnosis is beneficial or not and how to go about getting a diagnosis when it is felt one is needed. Topics are initially quite child-centred but gradually can become more relational when, for example, 'family scripts' get discussed.

The family school in London names a particular theme each month, which is used to organize lessons and other aspects of the school day. As an example, December was named the month when 'consideration for others' was highlighted. This lent itself well to a mentalization-focused parental learning session whereby material was presented which highlighted ways in which people can show, or fail to show, consideration for others. The parents explored this first and then engaged in a discussion about how their ideas might apply to their children and families. During the subsequent MFT session, the parents asked their children about their understanding of what it meant to 'consider others' and engaged their children in discussion. They then decided to go for an outing to a local market and for the children to demonstrate 'consideration for others' concretely by setting their children the task of buying an inexpensive item that would show consideration for another person.

Other family schools have different programmes. For example, the students at the family school in Cuxhaven (North Germany) are accompanied by a parent or a close adult caregiver for 3 days a week (see Box 13, Föhl & Tietjen, 2017). A typical day consists of a teaching program in the core subjects (e.g., mathematics, history) as well as multi-family work. The parents accompany the lessons in different ways, sometimes alongside their children, sometimes observing and sometimes via 'cross-fostering' of their respective children. While the children are in class, parent groups are held in parallel with specific parenting topics. In addition to their school goals, the children always work on daily goals that take into account their current difficulties. On the fourth day, the students attend the family school alone without their parents; they have formal lessons and also practice appropriate pro-social behaviour in joint cooperation exercises. On the fifth day, the students attend their mainstream school to work on their goals there and to get feedback from their ordinary school environment. This makes it clear to the children, the class and the teacher that the students still belong to the mainstream class and the school and that they are (still) welcome there.

Box 13   Timetable of Family School Cuxhaven
(Föhl & Tietjen, 2017)

Time	Themes
08:30–08:50	**Icebreaker activity** **Planning of daily goals**
08:50–09:35	**Lesson** Parents observe lesson from back of the class
09:35–09:45	**Break**
09:45–10:30	**Lesson** **Parallel parents' group**
10:30–10:45	**Pause**
10:45–12:00	**Multifamily activity**
12:00–12:30	**Final round** (reading of daily goals)

Weekly schedule

Monday	Tuesday	Wednesday	Thursday	Friday
Students and Parents	**Students and Parents**	**Students and Parents**	**Students**	**Students in mainstream school**

The family school in Berlin (Germany) offers 10 places for students with their families. The project is co-financed by the local social care and education departments (Beuth & Adolf, 2017). It is part of a mainstream school, separate but located on its school grounds so that the family school students use the same schoolyard with all the students attending the mainstream school. Embedded in the everyday life of a mainstream school, the Berlin family school is a complex yet 'realistic' context, which also helps parents to keep in touch with the reality of schooling. New families join viewing the family school first, without the practitioners being present, talking to other families about their experiences in and with the family school. A school network meeting is then called, and clear behavioural goals for the child are made, as well as goals for the parents. What is important right from the start is the close and mandatory involvement of the mainstream school, as the child remains a student there and attends it for 1 whole day per week (see the weekly schedule in Figure 10.1), thereby keeping in touch with the familiar network of friends and teachers.

In another family school, this time in Denmark (Hjordt et al., 2017), practitioners work with a total of 15 families, consisting of students age 6 to 15 and their parents. Parents and children attend 2 days a week from 8:30 a.m. to 12 p.m. One day a week, only the parents attend, from 8:30 a.m. to 12:30 p.m.

Time	Monday	Tuesday	Wednesday	Thursday	Friday
8.00–8.45	Icebreaker Planning of weekly goals	Lesson	Students in mainstream school all day	Lesson	Lesson
8.55–9.40	Lesson	Lesson		Lesson	Lesson
	Break	Break		Break	Break
10.00–10.45	Lesson		Team meeting		Lesson
10.00–11.15		MFT activity		Music therapy	
10.55–12.10	MFT activity		Supervision		MFT activity
11.25–12.10		Lesson		Lesson	
	Lunch	Lunch		Lunch	Lunch
12.30–13.30	Remedial teaching Single-family sessions	Remedial teaching Single-family sessions	Home visits until 16.00	Remedial teaching Single-family sessions	Remedial teaching Single-family sessions

Figure 10.1 Weekly schedule: Family School Berlin

Navigating the challenges of MFT in school settings

It is a sad fact that socially deprived children are more likely to struggle at school. It is also a sad fact that if their parents are employed, they are less likely to have jobs that are flexible enough for them to be able to attend a family class once weekly for a whole term – and they are even less likely to attend a family school for a whole day or more. Socially marginalized families are also less likely to have childcare for any pre-school children and hence will find participating in a family class or family school very challenging. In two-parent families, it may be possible for the parents to alternate attending the projects, but this is obviously not possible for one-parent families. Here sometimes a centrally involved grandparent or aunt/ uncle may attend some of the sessions in place of the parent. Whilst students could experience attendance at a family class in a mainstream school as being stigmatizing, our experience has been that this is rarely the case. In fact, it is not uncommon for other students to become curious about the project and request to attend as well. Here, however, it proves difficult to recruit those students' parents.

Chapter 11

Problem corner

Managing challenges – what to do if and when . . . ?

Managing typical problem scenarios

MFT practitioners regularly encounter typical, if not predictable, problems when working in a multi-family setting. Possible ways of managing these problems are described in this chapter. When practitioners first start to practice MFT and become acquainted with a new therapeutic modality, issues of technical mastery tend to be in the foreground. After some time, they begin to feel more comfortable with the model and start working a bit more flexibly. Trainee MFT practitioners usually go through five phases of what could be termed their 'professional journey', which is rife with pitfalls when trying to grasp MFT. In stage 1 budding practitioners experiment with a range of MFT activities, not really knowing why they choose some but not others. During the second phase they try to adapt the MFT activities to suit what they believe are the families' needs and therefore consider a range of alternative activities. The third phase is characterized by the introduction of some form of reflection to challenge stuck patterns. It is only during the fourth phase that practitioners-in-training will consider transferring substantial amounts of MFT skills outside the group. In phase 5 consideration is given to experimenting with different contextual settings during each session, including single-family, parental couple or even individual meetings. As trainees navigate these phases, they increasingly focus less on actual technique(s) and more on providing opportunities for families to self-manage the diverse therapeutic contexts.

However, as with other forms of therapy, problems that affect individuals, relationships or group cohesion, as well as with the framework itself, can surface. Several factors contribute to these: group pressure, challenges to do with the activities, intensification of interactions and resulting high level of arousal, emotional strain, fear of being 'infected' by the perceived 'ills' of other families and so on. Most practitioners understand that they are likely to witness strong emotions and crisis situations when undertaking MFT, and they will be anxious about how to deal with these. Whether these difficulties should be 'fixed' by the practitioners or whether the responsibility for doing so should be handed to group members is a dilemma that is often encountered.

DOI: 10.4324/9781003442424-11

When practitioners start their first MFT groups, it is important that they determine beforehand the activities that are going to take place during the project. They need to have preparation time to plan the project and to consider both content and timing of sessions. This can be done by drawing up a plan which sets out:

1. the general theme and sub-themes of each session;
2. the precise timings of each activity;
3. title and instructions for each activity;
4. the type of sub-groups planned;
5. the role(s) of each team member to avoid confusion during sessions.

It may well be the case that the families are not motivated, being neither proactive nor responsive, or indeed interested in the activities. Indeed, some of the first activities may not correspond to the needs of families at that time. In this case, it is useful to take a short break and to discuss with the coworker what possible solutions can be found to manage the seeming mismatch and avoid continuing at all costs. There are several possibilities: different sub-groups can be set up to carry out an activity; a speed-dating could be done with one of the questions being: '*How does this activity provide ideas for thinking about the issue of . . . ?*'; or one simply can start with a new activity. If the practitioners are unable to bounce back from the situation and cannot find a way out, the practitioners can discuss their dilemma in front of the families in a self-reflective conversation and ask the families for some helpful input.

Reviews involving all team members and associated professionals at the end of an MFT project are essential, focusing on positives and problematic situations, re-examining the themes, activities and previously made plans. Input from families can be sought through focus groups to get their feedback on what is and was useful or not. Over time, practitioners often add an 'alternatives folder' to their session plan so that they can respond more flexibly when something doesn't work.

In the following we have sub-divided typical challenges encountered during MFT into three categories: relational issues, participation issues and symptom-/problem-oriented issues. References to activities described in Chapter 6 are in cursive script (e.g., *Circle Game, Remote Control*).

A. Relational issues

A 1 Conflict between two (or more) adults

Scenario: Two parents get into an argument during an activity; other group members, including children, are getting upset.

Practitioners' response:

Any conflict that is at risk of escalation should be 'noticed and named' and then be put on halt. The practitioners can then propose the formation of two groups: one for the children and one for the adults. The adult group gets subdivided into small sub-groups of three adults each, with the two (or more) adults in conflict being placed in mere observer positions, listening to the sub-groups in turn. The sub-groups are asked to brainstorm about how to manage and resolve this conflict and consider its impact on the children. The ideas from each sub-group are presented, and, once all the adults are together, they design a message they will give to the children when both groups meet. Parents can also leave the room briefly with one of the team members to debrief and to identify ways of refocusing on the children's needs.

A 2 Conflict between children

Scenario: Two or more children get into a physical or verbal argument.

Practitioners' response:

Make the parents of each child responsible for down-regulating and emotionally containing their own child(ren) first. The unaffected parents and their children are encouraged to talk about their experiences and share strategies of managing conflicts between children and to then think about examples of reparation. During these discussions, the affected families remain in an observer position.

A 3 Threats or acts of physical violence from adults

Scenario: Adult being verbally aggressive to or physically chastising a child.

Practitioners' response:

Intervene immediately to protect child (guideline: 'child protection first, therapy second'). One practitioner can leave the room with the aggressive parent whilst the affected child is left in the care of the other practitioner or a suitable adult group member. Appropriate child protection measures need to be considered, including involvement of social services. Other parents may also need to be helped to down-regulate their arousal so that they are able to consider their children's needs.

A 4 Verbal abuse

Scenario: During an activity, there is an incident which leads to exchanges of verbal abuse, involving both adults and children.

Practitioners' response:

Reduce arousal by requesting everyone to be totally '*silent for 2 minutes and let the silence speak*'. Form single-family groups and ask them to identify ways of resolving the conflict that provoked the verbal abuse. Get families to share their ideas and then replay the scene that led to the conflict, freeze-framing the interactions at crucial points and inviting group members to mentalize the participants at each of those, considering the potential steps that could be taken to have a different outcome. If the child's and/or parent's level of arousal remains, it is best to leave the room with them to facilitate down-regulation prior to them joining the group again.

A 5 Discriminatory remarks

Scenario: Group member(s) discriminating against other(s) because of faith, disability, ethnicity, gender, age and so on.

Practitioners' response:

Form small sub-groups (three to four persons), which discuss what it may be like for someone in general – *not* the discriminated group member(s) – to be subjected to being discriminated against and ask them to explicitly mentalize *a* victimized person. Get each subgroup to feed back their ideas to the rest of the group, and then get sub-groups to put forward three 'rules' about what to do when prejudiced remarks are being made or discriminatory behaviours are displayed.

A 6 High-conflict post-separation between parents

Scenario: Parents who are separated and in a continuing high-conflict relationship enact these in the group.

Practitioners' response:

Establish with each parent, prior to them starting MFT, whether it is emotionally and physically safe for them to be in the same room and whether they can focus on their child(ren) rather than on their ex-partner or on the ongoing conflicts. If they are not able to do so, consideration will need to be given for them attending MFT in sequence (alternate sessions) rather than together. If the parents agree to attend together, the focus has to be on protecting the child(ren) from their conflicts and on parental cooperation. This may need to be re-emphasized at regular intervals throughout the MFT project. If parental cooperation is thought to be a possibility, a discussion can be proposed to sub-groups of parents on: 'the best recipes for successful parental cooperation'. A related experiential task can be given to the parents in conflict: to draw up the main rules for parental cooperation by *Moving the Pen with Four Hands*. This involves both parents holding the same pen and trying to write the rules on a sheet of paper.

A 7 Marginalization of a family

Scenario: One family is excluded or excludes themselves.

Practitioners' response:

Consider using the *Circle Game* activity. Also consider *Slow Speed-Dating* with getting people to talk about experiences of having felt excluded or of not having been part of something they had wanted to be part of. Then invite them to speak about what thoughts and feelings that has provoked in them. Finally group members can be asked to tell stories of how they overcame their marginalization.

A 8 One parent undermining a partner parent or carer

Scenario: A foster carer or parent undermines another parent/carer regarding their parenting of a child.

Practitioners' response:

Consider a role play with children acting as 'parents' who criticize each other over the head of a parent playing a child. In a debriefing group, members are asked what they think might be going on in the heart and mind of the child.

A 9 Safeguarding disclosure

Scenario: Practitioners and/or group members are concerned about the risk of abuse or neglect of a child.

Practitioners' response:

Assess the physical and emotional risks by seeing the child on their own. Discuss safety issues with the child's primary carers. Involve social services if the risk is deemed considerable. Involve adult group members in discussions and obtain advice from them.

A 10 Sibling conflict under the radar

Scenario: Physical fights/bullying between siblings gets ignored.

Practitioners' response:

Share your observations in the large group setting. Make the parent(s) of the siblings responsible for down-regulating and emotionally containing their children first. Encourage the other families to talk about their experiences of sibling conflicts, both from their own childhoods and currently, and get them to share strategies of managing sibling conflicts.

B. Participation issues

B 1 Different priorities

Scenario: During the task of choosing the first theme to be discussed, no agreement can be reached between families.

Practitioners' response:

Write the themes on which there is disagreement on large sheets of paper, place them in different parts of the room and get the group members to place themselves on the sheet of their choice. Suggest a sequence of how to address the themes, staring with the one that the majority of group members have chosen.

B 2 Excessive noise levels

Scenario: Very noisy and disruptive children.

Practitioners' response:

Make the parents responsible for managing their children to first create some quiet. The *Remote Control* activity can be employed. Alternatively, consider the 'beast taming' task which can be introduced as follows: '*Can all the children stand in a line? We want to see which family wins, and therefore we want each parent to whisper something in the ears of their child(ren). Who is going to be the winner and best at 'taming' their child? And then let us know a bit later what you whispered'.*

B 3 Silent group members

Scenario: One or more group members is unable/unwilling to talk in large or small group meetings.

Practitioners' response:

Respect the silence for the first two to three meetings, then suggest using a 'translator' – volunteer group member – the silent person whispers into his ear, with their voice then being amplified by the 'translator'. Consider asking the silent person to write down what they cannot say. To dramatize the situation, the piece of paper can be placed in a bottle, together with messages from other group members. The bottle can then be passed around, and one person can then pull out all the messages and reads them out.

B 4 Family member monopolizing the group

Scenario: One parent talks repetitively about their life and/or views, dominating the group.

Practitioners' response:

Response 1: Suggest limited talking time for everyone, such as 2 minutes maximum, '*So that everyone has got a fair chance*', with a bell signalling when time is up in extreme cases.

Response 2: Set up a *Speed-Dating* activity to collect ideas about the issue or theme the concerned adult had spoken so much about: '*What the parent talked about is a very emotional theme. Can each person in the speed-dating talk about any of their own experiences relating to this?*' These experiences can be collected afterwards and reflected upon in the larger group.

B 5 Persistent late-comers

Scenario: One or more families almost always arrive late.

Practitioners' response:

Start the meeting on time so that the rest of the group does not feel penalized. The impact of latecomers can be managed by beginning every meeting with an ice-breaker activity which latecomers can join without being stigmatized. A rota system can be installed, with each family – including the persistent latecomers – having in turn the task of introducing a group activity, with a maximum duration of 15 minutes.

B 6 Mobile phones and social media

Scenario: Parents or practitioners discover that during MFT posts members – and especially adolescents – are using mobile phones, sending tweets or involved in other forms of using social media.

Practitioners' response:

Response 1: Convene speed-dating for group members to discuss pros and cons of the use of mobile phones in the group. Collect a few ideas and then form small 'working parties' with the task of setting out rules for the use of mobile phones and social media during the group. Follow this up by asking each family task to devise five rules for the use of mobile phone and social media in their respective homes.

Response 2: Divide the group into three sub-groups (preferably avoiding parents being with their own children) and get them to think about three questions: How does social media contribute to socialization and self-esteem? How can social media create and heal problems? How can social media be used to combat the influence of problems? The three sub-groups can each draw up a manual on the use of social media during MFT sessions.

B 7 Badly matched families

Scenario: Families state that they have little in common and that they are just too different.

Practitioners' response:

Focus on non-problem issues and on what likes, interests, tastes and experiences different families and their individual members have in common. Consider activities like *Who Has Once . . .?* or *Finding Your Place.* An alternative is to use one family who feels very different as either co-facilitators or as official observers of the activity. They can then in a fishbowl setting discuss what they find different and why and what their observations were.

B 8 Reluctant attenders

Scenario: Parents or adolescents are reluctant to attend MFT sessions.

Practitioners' response:

Form small sub-groups which discuss the reasons why families or some of their members – but *not* the actual family, parents or adolescent – might be reluctant to attend MFT. Then get each sub-group to put forward strategies to motivate them and ask whether anyone might volunteer to implement some of the strategies. As to managing reluctant adolescents: consider allowing them to be in an adjoining room and appoint a 'messenger' who comes to report on what they are doing and inform them of what is happening in the large group.

B 9 Non-attendance/drop-out

Scenario: One family no longer attends.

Practitioners' response:

Get group members to devise a message to the family. Consider how and by whom the message is transmitted. If only one family member has dropped out, encourage the remaining members of that family to continue attending.

B 10 Family not able to complete an activity

Scenario: Family members are unable to start or finish a single-family activity (e.g., *Family Portrait, Mind Scan*).

Practitioners' response:

Invite other group members to assist and inspire the struggling family. Ask the members of the family in difficulty to look at what other families are doing. Encourage families to present the work they have done, even if it is incomplete, framing it as 'work in progress'.

B 11 Group member(s) refusing to participate in activities

Scenario: One or more group members find a proposed activity 'silly'.

Practitioners' response:

Validate the person's doubts and get other group members to talk in pairs and speculate what the purpose of the activity might be all about. In the likely scenario that there are mixed responses, divide the group in two, with one group engaging in the activity and the other more sceptical group members thinking of other ways of addressing the theme the activity is focusing on. If it is just one person, consider including them in the professional team as a 'conscientious objector' so that they can attend the activity, reflect with the professionals during the activity and conduct an interview with the families afterwards, supported by a professional.

B 12 No time to finish an activity

Scenario: Time does not permit for a specific activity to be completed and/or there is no time for reflecting.

Practitioners' response:

Provide brief bullet points of themes and issues and get group members to think about these '*between now and next time we meet*'. Ensure that the bullet points are referred to at the beginning of the next MFT meeting. One can also consider transforming the unfinished task into a collaborative moment: in randomly assigned sub-groups, group members have 5 minutes to find creative ways to preserve the unfinished activity, maybe by taking a photograph or by deciding whether, how or when to take it up – or just leave it.

B 13 Practitioners being too central

Scenario: Practitioners appear to do all the work and dominate the group.

Practitioners' response:

Address the families: '*We notice we talk too much, and we give too much advice. This must stop! It takes all agency away from you. We are going to leave the room now for 15 minutes, and when we get back, we would like to be surprised of how you organize yourselves in our absence*'. Another possibility is to choose from among the group members one or two 'co-workers' who can be used as a reflecting team, meta-communicating about the centrality of the practitioners. The co-workers can also be asked to interview other group members about the impasse: '*Can you and you interview that group over there while I interview this one?*'

B 14 Competing needs

Scenario: High levels of need in the group leads to parents competing for talking space.

Practitioners' response:

Notice and name the needs and invite ideas how the space can be shared to provide reassurance. Stick to timings and keep each person's contribution to no longer 2 or 3 minutes. Consider the possibility of 10-minute single sessions for a needy parent but remember to challenge them on how they manage their children in the meantime.

B 15 Different levels of engagement in an activity

Scenario: Some parents are really engaged in the group work; others are not.

Practitioners' response:

Use motivated group members to help the less keen members.

B 16 Practitioners feel self-conscious or silly

Scenario: Events in group appear to undermine the practitioners.

Practitioners' response:

Only use activities you feel you can facilitate with some confidence. Discuss with your co-practitioner to identify any potential underlying personal issues you may have around an activity. When a problem arises and you feel uncomfortable, interrupt the activity and organize discussions in pairs or small subgroups to understand the sequence of events. Be humble and acknowledge that you may have chosen the wrong activity for this group.

B 17 Outside professional wants to attend session

Scenario: A family asks that a professional who cares for their child in another service wants to come to the group 'to understand what this is all about'.

Practitioners' response:

Consider asking all group members to think about the issue and for them to state what they feel about the request. Follow this up by asking whether any of the other families would want to invite professionals and get families to the pros and cons, as well as what the purpose might be in this particular case. If other families also ask for professionals who are involved with them to attend MFT, get the families to plan and organize this as a one-off event.

B 18 Families are very literal and/or concrete

Scenario: A parent or adolescent remain stuck in a concrete description of their problem and find it difficult to mentalize themselves and others.

Practitioners' response:

Consider dramatizing mentalizing processes by using props, like white coats for adolescents, and state: '*Here you are doctors, and you must think about the problem of this family*'. Then provide large pens and notebooks for the parents, and state: '*And you are journalists in the middle of an investigation to understand how this family works*', and provide special glasses and a stethoscope for two other group members, and state: '*You are experts who must solve this problem*'. Family members are then interviewed while remaining in their respective roles.

B 21 'I don't know' responses

Scenario: During a group discussion, a teenager responds to each request with '*I don't know*' or shoulder shrugging.

Practitioners' response:

Consider forming subgroups, each having to address the question: '*How many different ideas can we express when we only have one sentence?*' Examples are provided and shared. This is followed by everyone to join for a competition about all the possibilities of what 'I don't know' (or shoulder shrugging) might mean. Each team is composed of three or four people and has to the tone of voice, loudness and speed of delivery of 'I don't know'. What all the different 'I don't knows' mean has to be described in subtitles and the team with the most subtitles wins. If asked what the prize is, practitioners can reply 'I don't know'.

C. Issues related to symptoms or problems

C 1 Withdrawn adolescents

Scenario: Adolescents do not participate in activities or absent themselves.

Practitioners' response:

Accept and do not challenge the adolescent during the first few MFT sessions. Consider involving peers to connect with the young person in a 1:1 context. Consider using the *Circle Game* activity. Also consider organizing a discussion in small teams to reflect on what might be hindering a young person's participation.

C 2 Contamination fears

Scenario: Parents are afraid that the presence of group members with challenging or 'abnormal' behaviours can negatively influence their own children.

Practitioners' response:
Initiate a discussion, in sub-groups of three to four persons, about how a problem can threaten to colonize a group, focusing on how to manage the threat and to protect oneself, based on past experiences. Get feedback, then name the 'problem' (e.g., eating disorder, aggressive behaviour, suicidality) and get the same sub-groups to discuss how the challenging group members are similar and different from a virus and how one can limit or counter its influence, including identifying warning signs.

C 3 Profuse displays of emotions and anxieties

Scenario: A parent bursts into tears, hyperventilates and/or leaves room in visible distress.
Practitioners' response:
First encourage group members to see what they can do to help the parent. Practitioners to focus on protecting the child(ren) from being exposed to their parent's distress, including taking them away from the scene of distress, such as into another room.
Divide the group into sub-groups and get each to think about what might have happened to the parent. Then focus the discussion on the advantages and disadvantages of a parent of showing their emotions to their child and talking about them. Finally, each sub-group designs a message that can be delivered to the child.

C 4 Suicidal talk and behaviour

Scenario: Young person says during or at the end of an activity that they want to end their life.
Practitioners' response:
Undertake a brief risk assessment of the young person and make plans/take action to protect them if this is required. Form separate parents' and children's groups and get the parents to exchange ideas about how to manage such an announcement. Invite the children/young persons in their group to put forward *'dreams about a better life'* and what would need to happen to make the dream become reality.

C 5 Suspicion of group member being under the influence of alcohol/drugs

Scenario: Group member is inebriated or behaves as if on drugs.
Practitioners' response:
Challenge the group member in a private conversation and temporarily exclude them from participating in MFT that day. Announce to the group that the person concerned will not be able to participate that day. State that it is up to the person to explain their absence if they wish to. If it concerns a parent who is the sole carer for their child(ren), social services may need to be contacted.

C 6 Inappropriate adult conversations in front of children

Scenario: Two or more adults are engaged in a conversation which would seem to be inappropriate for children to be exposed to, in terms of content and/or the children's developmental stages.

Practitioners' response:

Create separate groups if content or level of conversations are not appropriate for children. Focus on parental impact awareness. Ask parents' group to think about what should be said to the children, taking into account the children's developmental stages and needs. Consider a five-step intervention along the lines of '*We notice that you are having an interesting conversation, but your children are left to their own devices; what do you think is going on in their heads?*'

C 7 Child being persistently abusive to parent

Scenario: A child physically and/or verbally attacks parent(s). A teenager insults his parent and pushes them aside violently.

Practitioners' response:

Consider convening a parents' group with a focus on why *a* child might behave the way they do. Get parents to share their respective experiences, recent and past, including in their own family of origin, and invite them to design strategies to manage similar future situations. In the children's group, they can be asked to imagine how it feels to see one's parent belittled or physically hurt by a loved one.

Chapter 12

Looking back and looking ahead . . .

Multi-family groups started informally in the waiting room of a mental hospital in New York in the late 1940s. Families with major issues in common saw something they recognized in one another. They started talking and made connections as they waited for their family member's psychosis to be treated by 'experts'. Those experts saw the therapeutic potential of bringing families with similar preoccupations and problems together, and multi-family therapy was born. MFT has since been developed to help families with a broad range of difficulties across many different service contexts all over the world. There are now core components of MFT that have been established for some time. These include de-centralizing the therapist, context making, promoting solidarity, stimulating fresh perspectives, strengthening reflectiveness, intensifying interactions, using feedback and experimentation and building on competencies. And the model continues to be refined, combining key concepts and techniques from systemic family therapy with mentalization-based approaches. Multifamily groups have always provided a natural context for the development and recovery of 'mentalizing', even before the term was coined. Yet the focus on enhancing effective mentalizing furthers the therapeutic potential of multi-family groups by facilitating more sophisticated context-making and providing additional techniques which align well with the systemic approach. Furthermore, the focus on mentalizing helps practitioners to have a more nuanced understanding of therapeutic processes and contributes to the creation of a setting where families feel safe, connected and thus open to social learning in ways that can be transferred to their lives outside of the group.

Research to date has provided generally positive results regarding the outcomes of multifamily therapy. Furthermore, there is very strong research linking social support and mental health (Harandi et al., 2017) and identifying the therapeutic alliance as a reliable predictor of good outcomes in therapy across different modalities (Martin et al., 2000; Baier et al., 2020). These findings are relevant because the experiences of connection and trust are thought to be key mechanisms of change in MFT. However, heterogeneity regarding treatment populations, treatment delivery and fidelity, as well as interactions with other treatments and interventions and issues with research methodology, have made it difficult to draw firm conclusions about the impact of MFT. Process research highlights factors such as

DOI: 10.4324/9781003442424-12

group cohesion and support, experiences of communality, learning by observation and experimentation, insight, hope, self-disclosure, high levels of satisfaction and adherence. These factors appear to map well onto the 'therapeutic ingredients' predicted by theories of change, but more research is needed.

In recent years there has been a substantial reported increase in people experiencing relational and mental health difficulties. Already stretched services are unable to keep up with the increasing demand in a financially pressured climate, and crucial opportunities to intervene early are missed while problems worsen and become more resistant to treatment. The cost to society increases when such difficulties impact employment, education and parenting. Most mental health needs in children and young people are unmet, with minoritized groups least likely to be helped (Patel et al., 2007, 2018). MFT could help with the problem of unmet need, as it uses the healing power of social connection to strengthen family systems and mental health in a live, natural and generalizable way. Whether it is delivered as an early or first-line intervention or as an adjunct to individual treatments, the fact that MFT employs the internal resources of the families that attend rather than the imposed resources of professional 'experts', and the fact that it can be easily delivered in the community, makes it a good 'fit' for families, including minoritized groups. As it is an approach that does not require practitioners to be highly specialist mental health professionals, MFT can be grown as a resource relatively quickly and inexpensively. All these factors make it an intervention that could extend the reach and effectiveness of existing services.

However, whilst versatility is a strength of MFT, it is also its weakness when it comes to demonstrating positive outcomes. To build the evidence base, there is a need for more systematic, rigorous research which describes the intervention delivered and pays attention to model fidelity and the interactions between MFT and other interventions. To be true to the principles of MFT, there is also a need for more systematic and explicit involvement of families in the development and delivery of the approach. One way forward is for MFT practitioners across the world to connect, co-ordinate and learn from each other in much the same way families are encouraged to do. Seasoned and aspiring multifamily practitioners can connect with each other by registering their interest at *multifamilyproject.org*.

References

Andersen, T. (1987) The reflecting team. *Family Process* 26, 415–428.

Asen, E. (1997) From Milan to Milan: True tales about the structural Milan approach. *Human Systems* 8, 39–42.

Asen, E. (2002) Multiple family therapy: An overview. *Journal of Family Therapy* 24, 3–16.

Asen, E. (2004) Collaborating in promiscuous swamps – the systemic practitioner as context chameleon? *Journal of Family Therapy* 26, 280–285.

Asen, E. (2007) Multi-contextual multiple family therapy. In: Mayes, L., Fonagy, P., & Target, M. (eds): *Developmental Science and Psychoanalysis*. London: Karnac.

Asen, E., Campbell, C., & Fonagy, P. (2019) Social systems: Beyond the microcosm of the individual and family. In: Bateman, A. W., & Fonagy, P. (eds.): *Handbook of Mentalizing in Mental Health Practice* (2nd ed., pp. 229–243). Washington, DC: American Psychiatric Publishing.

Asen, E., Dawson, N., & McHugh, B. (2001) *Multiple Family Therapy. The Marlborough Model and Its Wider Applications*. London & New York: Karnac.

Asen, E., & Fonagy, P. (2012a) Mentalization-based family therapy. In: Bateman, A., & Fonagy, P. (eds.): *Handbook of Mentalizing in Mental Health Practice* (pp. 107–128). Washington & London: American Psychiatric Publishing.

Asen, E., & Fonagy, P. (2012b) Mentalization-based therapeutic interventions for families. *Journal of Family Therapy* 34, 347–370.

Asen, E., & Fonagy, P. (2021) *Mentalization-Based Treatment with Families*. New York & London: Guilford Press.

Asen, E., & Morris, E. (2020) *High-Conflict Parenting Post-Separation: The Making and Breaking of Family Ties*. London: Routledge.

Asen, E., & Scholz, M. (2010) *Multi-Family Therapy: Concepts and Techniques*. London: Routledge.

Asen, E., & Scholz, M. (eds.). (2017) *Handbuch der Familientherapie*. Carl-Auer, Heidelberg.

Asen, E., & Schuff, H. (2006) Psychosis and multiple family group therapy. *Journal of Family Therapy* 28, 58–72.

Asen, E., Stein, R., Stevens, A., McHugh, B., Greenwood, J., & Cooklin, A. (1982) A day unit for families. *Journal of Family Therapy* 4, 345–358.

Asnaani, A. (2023) *A Cultural Humility and Social Justice Approach to Psychotherapy: Seven Applied Guidelines for Evidence-Based Practice*. Oxford: Oxford University Press.

Baier, A. L., Kline, A. C., & Feeny, N. C. (2020) Therapeutic alliance as a mediator of change: A systematic review and evaluation of research. *Clinical Psychology Review* 82, 101921.

Bansal, N., Karlsen, S., Sashidharan, S. P., Cohen, R., Chew-Graham, C. A., & Malpass, A. (2022) Understanding ethnic inequalities in mental healthcare in the UK: A meta-ethnography. *PLoS Medicine* 19(12), e1004139.

Baudinet, J., Eisler, I., Dawson, L., Simic, M., & Schmidt, U. (2021) Multi-family therapy for eating disorders: A systematic scoping review of the quantitative and qualitative findings. *International Journal of Eating Disorders* 54(12), 2095–2120.

Baudinet, J., Eisler, I., Konstantellou, A., Hunt, T., Kassamali, F., McLaughlin, N., Simic, M., & Schmidt, U. (2023) Perceived change mechanisms in multi-family therapy for anorexia nervosa: A qualitative follow-up study of adolescent and parent experiences. *European Eating Disorders Review* 31(6), 822–836.

Beuth, S., & Adolf, C. (2017) Familienschule in der Grossstadt. In: Asen, E., & Scholz, M. (eds.): *Handbuch der Familientherapie* (pp. 326–332). Heidelberg: Carl-Auer.

Binns, A., & Cardy, J. (2019) Developmental social pragmatic interventions for preschoolers with autism spectrum disorder: A systematic review. *Autism and Developmental Language Impairments* 4(1), 1–18.

Bishop, P., Clilverd, A., Cooklin, A., & Hunt, U. (2002) Mental health matters: A multi-family framework for mental health interventions. *Journal of Family Therapy* 24, 31–45.

Burnham, J. (2018) Developments in social GRRRAAACCEEESSS: Visible – invisible and voiced – unvoiced 1. In: *Culture and Reflexivity in Systemic Psychotherapy* (pp. 139–160). London: Routledge.

Byrne, S. M., & McLean, N. J. (2002) The cognitive-behavioral model of bulimia nervosa: A direct evaluation. *International Journal of Eating Disorders* 31(1), 17–31.

Byrne, G., Sleed, M., Midgley, N., Fearon, P., Mein, C., Bateman, A., & Fonagy, P. (2019) Lighthouse parenting programme: Description and pilot evaluation of mentalization-based treatment to address child maltreatment. *Clinical Child Psychology and Psychiatry* 24(4), 680–693.

Campion, J., Bhugra, D., Bailey, S., & Marmot, M. (2013) Inequality and mental disorders: Opportunities for action. *The Lancet* 382(9888), 183–184.

Casey, P., Patalay, P., Deighton, J., Miller, S. D., & Wolpert, M. (2020) The child outcome rating scale: Validating a four-item measure of psychosocial functioning in community and clinic samples of children aged 10–15. *European Child & Adolescent Psychiatry* 29, 1089–1102.

Cecchin, G. (1987) Hypothesising, circularity and neutrality revisited: An invitation to curiosity. *Family Process* 26, 405–413.

Cook-Darzens, S., Gelin, Z., & Hendrick, S. (2018) Evidence base for multiple family therapy (MFT) in non-psychiatric conditions and problems: A review (part 2). *Journal of Family Therapy* 40(3), 326–343.

Cooklin, A. (2006) Children as carers of parents with mental illness. *Psychiatry* 5(1), 32–35.

Cooklin, A., Bishop, P., Francis, D., Fagin, L., & Asen, E. (2011) *The Kidstime Workshops – A Social Intervention for the Children of Parents with Mental Illness and Their Parents*. London: CAMHS Publications.

Cooklin, A., Miller, A., & McHugh, B. (1983) An institution for change: Developing a family day unit. *Family Process* 22, 453–468.

Cronen, V. E., Barnett, P. W., & Harris, L. M. (1979) The logic of the coordinated management of meaning: A rules-based approach to the first course in interpersonal communication. *Communication Education* 28, 22–38. doi: 10.1080/03634527909378327.

Dare, C., & Eisler, I. (2000) A multi-family group day treatment programme for adolescent eating disorder. *European Eating Disorders Review* 8, 4–18.

Davis, D. E., DeBlaere, C., Owen, J., Hook, J. N., Rivera, D. P., Choe, E., Van Tongeren, D. R., Worthington, E. L., Jr., & Placeres, V. (2018) The multicultural orientation framework: A narrative review. *Psychotherapy* 55(1), 89–100. doi: 10.1037/pst0000160.

Dawson, N., & McHugh, B. (1994) Parents and children: Participants in change. In: Dowling, E., & Osborne, E. (eds.): *The Family and the School: A Joint Systems Approach to Problems with Children*. London: Routledge.

Eisler, I., Simic, M., Hodsoll, J., Asen, E., Berelowitz, M., Connan, F., Ellis, G., Hugo, P., Schmidt, U., Treasure, J., & Yi, I. (2016) A pragmatic randomised multi-centre trial of multifamily and single family therapy for adolescent anorexia nervosa. *BMC Psychiatry* 16, 1–14.

Engman-Bredvik, S., & Suarez, N. C. (2016) Multi-family therapy in anorexia nervosa: A qualitative study of parental experiences. In *Innovations in Family Therapy for Eating Disorders* (pp. 262–274). Routledge.

Föhl, M., & Tietjen, O. (2017) Familienschule im ländlichen Raum. In: Asen, E., & Scholz, M. (eds.): *Handbuch der Familientherapie* (pp. 314–325). Heidelberg: Carl-Auer.

Fonagy, P., & Luyten, P. (2009) A developmental, mentalization-based approach to the understanding and treatment of borderline personality disorder. *Development and Psychopathology* 21, 1355–1381.

Fonagy, P., Luyten, P., & Allison, E. (2015) Epistemic petrification and the restoration of epistemic trust: A new conceptualization of borderline personality disorder and its psychosocial treatment. *Journal of Personality Disorders* 29, 575–609.

Fonagy, P., Steele, M., Steele, H., Moran, G. S., & Higgitt, A. C. (1991) The capacity for understanding mental states: The reflective self in parent and child and its significance for security of attachment. *Infant Mental Health Journal* 12(3), 201–218.

Foulkes, S. H. (1948) *Group-Analytic Psychotherapy*. Reprinted 1983, London: Karnac Books.

Fraenkel, P. (2006) Engaging families as experts: Collaborative family program development. *Family Process* 45, 237–257.

Gallotti, M., & Frith, C. D. (2013) Social cognition in the we-mode. *Trends in Cognitive Sciences* 17, 160–165.

Gelin, Z., Cook-Darzens, S., & Hendrick, S. (2018) The evidence base for multiple family therapy in psychiatric disorders: A review (part 1). *Journal of Family Therapy* 40(3), 302–325.

Gelin, Z., Cook-Darzens, S., Simon, Y., & Hendrick, S. (2016) Two models of multiple family therapy in the treatment of adolescent anorexia nervosa: A systematic review. *Eating and Weight Disorders-Studies on Anorexia, Bulimia and Obesity* 21, 19–30.

Goodman, R. (2001) Psychometric properties of the strengths and difficulties questionnaire. *Journal of the American Academy of Child & Adolescent Psychiatry* 40(11), 1337–1345.

Grácio, J., Gonçalves-Pereira, M., & Leff, J. (2016) What do we know about family interventions for psychosis at the process level? A systematic review. *Family Process* 55(1), 79–90.

Hall, E. T. (1976) *Beyond Culture*. New York: Anchor Press.

Harandi, T. F., Taghinasab, M. M., & Nayeri, T. D. (2017) The correlation of social support with mental health: A meta-analysis. *Electronic Physician* 9(9), 5212.

Hays, P. A. (2008) *Addressing Cultural Complexities in Practice: Assessment, Diagnosis, & Therapy* (2nd ed.). Washington, DC: American Psychological Association.

Hazel, N. A., McDonell, M. G., Short, R. A., Berry, C. M., Voss, W. D., Rodgers, M. L., & Dyck, D. G. (2004) Impact of multiple-family groups for outpatients with schizophrenia on caregivers' distress and resources. *Psychiatric Services* 55(1), 35–41.

Hellemans, S., De Mol, J., Buysse, A., Eisler, I., Demyttenaere, K., & Lemmens, G. M. D. (2011) Therapeutic processes in multi-family groups for major depression: Results of an interpretative phenomenological study. *Journal of Affective Disorders* 134(1–3), 226–234.

Hertzmann, L., Target, M., Hewison, D., Casey, P., Fearon, P., & Lassri, D. (2016) Mentalization-based therapy for parents in entrenched conflict: A random allocation feasibility study. *Psychotherapy* 53(4), 388.

Hjordt, T., Christensen, P. V., Cadan., E. G., Rasmussen, T., Strand, A., & Wilson, H. (2017) Mentalisierungsinspirierte Arbeit an einer dänischen Familienschule. In: Asen, E., & Scholz, M. (eds.): *Handbuch der Familientherapie* (pp. 33–345). Heidelberg: Carl-Auer.

Jewell, T., & Lemmens, G. (2018) Multiple family therapy: Forever promising? Commentary on Gelin et al. (2018) and Cook-Darzens et al. (2018), the evidence base for multiple family therapy in psychiatric and non-psychiatric conditions: A review (parts 1 and 2). *Journal of Family Therapy* 40(3), 344–348.

Kanner, L. (1943) Autistic disturbances of affective contact. *Nervous Child* 2(3), 217–250.

Laqueur, H. P., Laburt, H. A., & Morong, E. (1964) Multiple family therapy. *Current Psychiatric Therapies* 4, 150–154.

Lemmens, G. M., Eisler, I., Dierick, P., Lietaer, G., & Demyttenaere, K. (2009) Therapeutic factors in a systemic multi-family group treatment for major depression: Patients' and partners' perspectives. *Journal of Family Therapy* 31(3), 250–269.

Lemmens, G. M., Wauters, S., Heireman, M., Eisler, I., Lietaer, G., & Sabbe, B. (2003) Beneficial factors in family discussion groups of a psychiatric day clinic: perceptions by the therapeutic team and the families of the therapeutic process. *Journal of Family Therapy* 25(1), 41–63.

Ma, J. L. C., Lai, K. Y. C., & Wan, E. S. F. (2017) Multifamily group intervention for Chinese parents and their children with attention deficit hyperactivity disorder in a Chinese context. *Social Work with Groups* 40, 244–260.

Ma, J. L. C., Lai, K. Y. C., & Xia, L. L. (2018) Treatment efficacy of multiple family therapy for Chinese families of children with attention deficit hyperactivity disorder. *Family Process* 57, 399–414.

Martin, D. J., Garske, J. P., & Davis, M. K. (2000) Relation of the therapeutic alliance with outcome and other variables: A meta-analytic review. *Journal of Consulting and Clinical Psychology* 68(3), 438.

Marty, P. (1991) *Mentalisation et psychomatique*. Paris: Laborataire Delagrange.

Mason, B. (2019) Re-visiting safe uncertainty: Six perspectives for clinical practice and the assessment of risk. *Journal of Family Therapy* 41, 343–356.

McCrory, E. J., & Viding, E. (2015) The theory of latent vulnerability: Reconceptualizing the link between childhood maltreatment and psychiatric disorder. *Development and Psychopathology* 27(2), 493–505.

McDonell, M. G., Short, R. A., Hazel, N. A., Berry, C. M., & Dyck, D. G. (2006) Multiple-family group treatment of outpatients with schizophrenia: Impact on service utilization. *Family Process* 45(3), 359–373.

McFarlane, W. R. (2016) Family interventions for schizophrenia and the psychoses: A review. *Family Process* 55(3), 460–482.

McFarlane, W. R., Dunne, E., Lukens, E., Deakins, S., Horen, B., Newmark, M., & McLaughlin-Toran, J. (1993) From research to clinical practice: Dissemination of New York State's family psychoeducation project. *Psychiatric Services* 44(3), 265–270.

McFarlane, W. R., Link, B., Dushay, R., Marchal, J., & Crilly, J. (1995a) Psychoeducational multiple family groups: Four-year relapse outcome in schizophrenia. *Family Process* 34(2), 127–144.

McFarlane, W. R., Lukens, E., Link, B., Dushay, R., Deakins, S. A., Newmark, M., Dunne, E. J., Horen, B., & Toran, J. (1995b) Multiple-family groups and psychoeducation in the treatment of schizophrenia. *Archives of General Psychiatry* 52(8), 679–687.

Miller, S. D., Duncan, B. L., Brown, J., Sparks, J. A., & Claud, D. A. (2003) The outcome rating scale: A preliminary study of the reliability, validity, and feasibility of a brief visual analog measure. *Journal of Brief Therapy* 2(2), 91–100.

Minuchin, S. (1974) *Families and Family Therapy*. Cambridge, MA: Harvard University Press.

Morris, E. (2017) 'Early days' – Arbeit mit Eltern und Babys. In: Asen, E., & Scholz, M. (eds.): *Handbuch der Familientherapie* (pp. 166–174). Heidelberg: Carl-Auer.

Morris, E., Le Huray, C., Skagerberg, E., Gomes, R., & Ninteman, A. (2014) Families changing families: The protective function of multi-family therapy for children in education. *Clinical Child Psychology and Psychiatry* 19(4), 617–632.

Mueser, K. T., Salyers, M. P., & Mueser, P. R. (2001) A prospective analysis of work in schizophrenia. *Schizophrenia Bulletin* 27(2), 281–296.

Nashef, A., & Mohr, L. (2017) Kinder und Jugendliche mit einer Autismusspektrumstöung. In: Asen, E., & Scholz, M. (eds.): *Handbuch der Familientherapie* (pp. 105–115). Heidelberg: Carl-Auer.

Overbeek, M. M., Gudde, O. M., Rijnberg, C., Hempel, R., Beijer, D., & Maras, A. (2021/2023) Multi-problem families in intensive specialised multifamily therapy: Theoretical description and case report. *Journal of Family Therapy* 43, 81–93. doi: 10.1111/1467-6427.12320.

Owen, J., Tao, K. W., Imel, Z. E., Wampold, B. E., & Rodolfa, E. (2014) Addressing racial and ethnic microaggressions in therapy. *Professional Psychology: Research and Practice* 45(4), 283.

Owen, J. J., Tao, K., Leach, M. M., & Rodolfa, E. (2011) Clients' perceptions of their psychotherapists' multicultural orientation. *Psychotherapy* 48(3), 274.

Patel, V., Flisher, A. J., Hetrick, S., & McGorry, P. (2007) Mental health of young people: A global public-health challenge. *The Lancet* 369(9569), 1302–1313.

Patel, V., Saxena, S., Lund, C., Thornicroft, G., Baingana, F., Bolton, P., Chisholm, D., Collins, P. Y., Cooper, J. L., Eaton, J., Herrman, H., & Unützer, J. (2018) The Lancet Commission on global mental health and sustainable development. *The Lancet* 392(10157), 1553–1598.

Pérez-García, M., Sempere-Pérez, J., Rodado-Martínez, J. V., López, D. P., Llor-Esteban, B., & Jiménez-Barbero, J. A. (2020) Effectiveness of multifamily therapy for adolescent disruptive behavior in a public institution: A randomized clinical trial. *Children and Youth Services Review* 117, 105289.

Selvini Palazzoli, M., Boscolo, L., Cecchin, G., & Prata, G. (1980) Hypothesizing-circularity-neutrality; three guidelines for the conductor of the session. *Family Process* 19, 3–12.

Schemmel, H., Selig, D., & Janschewk-Schlesinger, R. (2008) *Kunst als Ressource in der Therapie*. Tübingen: Dgvt-Verlag.

Schmidt, U., & Asen, E. (2005) Does multi-family day treatment hit the spot that other treatments cannot reach. *Journal of Family Therapy* 27(2), 101–103.

Scholz, M., & Asen, E. (2001) Multiple family therapy with eating disordered adolescents: Concepts and preliminary results. *European Eating Disorders Review* 9, 33–42.

Simic, M., Baudinet, J., Blessitt, E., Wallis, A., & Eisler, I. (2023) *Multi-Family Therapy for Anorexia Nervosa. A Treatment Manual*. Abingdon & New York: Routledge.

Simic, M., & Eisler, I. (2015) Multi-family therapy. *Family Therapy for Adolescent Eating and Weight Disorders* 1, 110–138.

Stubbe, D. (2020) Practicing cultural competence and cultural humility in the care of diverse patients. *Focus* 18, 49–51. doi: 10.1176/appi.focus.20190041.

Tervalon, M., & Murray-Garcia, J. (1998) Cultural humility versus cultural competence: A critical distinction in defining physician training outcomes in multicultural education. *Journal of Health Care for the Poor and Underserved* 9(2), 117–125. doi: 10.1353/hpu.2010.0233.

Thomas, M. S., Crosby, S., & Vanderhaar, J. (2019) Trauma-informed practices in schools across two decades: An interdisciplinary review of research. *Review of Research in Education* 43(1), 422–452. doi: 10.3102/0091732X18821123.

Tomm, K. (1988) Interventive interviewing: Part III. Intending to ask lineal, circular, strategic and reflexive questions. *Family Process* 27, 1–15.

Tuomela, R. (2006) Joint intention, we-mode and I-mode. *Midwest Studies in Philosophy* 30, 35–58.

Valdez, C. R., Abegglen, J., & Hauser, C. T. (2013) Fortalezas familiares program: Building sociocultural and family strengths in Latina women with depression and their families. *Family Process* 52(3), 378–393.

Van Beek, Y., Hessen, D., Levelt, L., Beujer, S., Rijnberg, C., Maras, A., & Overbeek, M. M. (2023) Intensive specialised multi-family therapy for multi-stressed families: Therapeutic alliance as predictor for effectiveness. *Journal of Family Therapy* 45, 271–290.

van Es, C. M., El Khoury, B., van Dis, E. A., Te Brake, H., van Ee, E., Boelen, P. A., & Mooren, T. (2023) The effect of multiple family therapy on mental health problems and family functioning: A systematic review and meta-analysis. *Family Process* 62(2), 499–514.

Van Lawick, J., & Visser, M. (2015) No kids in the middle: Dialogical and creative work with parents and children in the context of high conflict divorce. *Australian and New Zealand Journal of Family Therapy* 6, 33–50.

Vaughn, C., & Leff, J. (1976) The measurement of expressed emotion in the families of psychiatric patients. *British Journal of Social and Clinical Psychology* 15(2), 157–165.

Visser, M., Finkenauer, C., Schoemaker, K., Kluwer, E., Rijken, R. V., Lawick, J. V., Bom, H., de Schipper, J. C., & Lamers-Winkelman, F. (2017) I'll never forgive you: High conflict divorce, social network, and co-parenting conflicts. *Journal of Child and Family Studies* 26(11), 3055–3066.

Visser, M., & Van Lawick, J. (2021) *Group Therapy for High-Conflict Divorce: The 'No Kids in the Middle' Intervention Program*. Abingdon: Routledge.

Volkert, J., Taubner, S., Byrne, G., Rossouw, T., & Midgley, N. (2022) Introduction to mentalization-based approaches for parents, children, youths, and families. *American Journal of Psychotherapy* 75(1), 4–11.

Voriadaki, T., Simic, M., Espie, J., & Eisler, I. (2015) Intensive multi-family therapy for adolescent anorexia nervosa: Adolescents' and parents' day-to-day experiences. *Journal of Family Therapy* 37(1), 5–23.

White, M. (1995) Reflecting teamwork as definitional ceremony. In: White, M. (ed.): *Re-Authoring Lives: Interviews and Essays*. Adelaide: Dulwich Centre.

White, M., & Epston, D. (1990) *Narrative Means to Therapeutic Ends*. New York: W. W. Norton.

Woolgar, M., Humayun, S., Scott, S., & Dadds, M. R. (2023) I know what to do; I can do it; it will work: The brief parental self efficacy scale (BPSES) for parenting interventions. *Child Psychiatry & Human Development*, 1–10.

Yalom, I. D., & Leszcz, M. (1995) The therapeutic factors. In: *The Theory and Practice of Group Psychotherapy* (pp. 70–101). New York: Basic Books.

Index